A Pocketbook Manual of Hand and Upper Extremity Anatomy

Primus Manus

A Pocketbook Manual of
Hand and Upper Extremity Anatomy
Primus Manus

Fraser J. Leversedge, MD
Assistant Professor
Department of Orthopaedic Surgery
Duke University
Durham, North Carolina

Charles A. Goldfarb, MD
Associate Professor
Department of Orthopaedic Surgery
Washington University School of Medicine
St Louis, Missouri

Martin I. Boyer, MD
Carole B. and Jerome T. Loeb Professor of Orthopaedic Surgery
Washington University School of Medicine
St Louis, Missouri

Illustrations by Michael Lin, MD, PhD

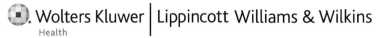
. Wolters Kluwer | Lippincott Williams & Wilkins
Health
Philadelphia · Baltimore · New York · London
Buenos Aires · Hong Kong · Sydney · Tokyo

Acquisitions Editor: Robert Hurley
Product Manager: Elise M. Paxson
Production Manager: Bridgett Dougherty
Senior Manufacturing Manager: Benjamin Rivera

Marketing Manager: Lisa Lawrence
Design Coordinator: Doug Smock
Production Service: MPS Limited, A Macmillan Company

© 2010 by LIPPINCOTT WILLIAMS & WILKINS, a WOLTERS KLUWER business
530 Walnut Street
Philadelphia, PA 19106 USA
LWW.com

Printed in The United States of America

Library of Congress Cataloging-in-Publication Data

Leversedge, Fraser J.
  A pocketbook of hand and upper extremity anatomy : *primus manus* / Fraser J. Leversedge, Charles A. Goldfarb, Martin I. Boyer ; illustrations by Michael Lin.—1st ed.
        p. ; cm.
  Includes bibliographical references and index.
  Summary: "Hand and upper extremity anatomy forms the basis of a comprehensive understanding of the physiology and pathologic conditions which influence function of the upper limb. Importantly, the intricate relationships and interactions between these diverse tissues define our unique capabilities for human function. The study of anatomy is analogous to the study of art; one must understand anatomy in order to appreciate it—in order to understand anatomy, however, one must appreciate its complexity of form and function, not withstanding its variations and anomalies. In an era where time spent in the anatomy laboratory has been de-emphasized within the medical education curriculum, an appreciation for anatomic relationships gained from a hands-on experience may suffer; a lack of awareness for anatomic detail may translate into the unfortunate consequence of a less detailed clinical assessment or a compromised treatment plan"—Provided by publisher.
  ISBN-13: 978-1-60831-466-9
  ISBN-10: 1-60831-466-9
1. Hand—Anatomy—Handbooks, manuals, etc. 2. Arm—Anatomy—Handbooks, manuals, etc.
  I. Goldfarb, Charles A. II. Boyer, Martin I. III. Title.
  [DNLM: 1. Upper Extremity—anatomy & histology—Handbooks. 2. Hand—anatomy & histology—Handbooks. WE 39 L661p 2010]
  QM548.L484 2010
  611'.97—dc22   2010021829

To purchase additional copies of this book, call our customer service department at (800) 638-3030 or fax orders to (301) 223-2320. International customers should call (301) 223-2300.

Visit Lippincott Williams & Wilkins on the Internet: at LWW.com. Lippincott Williams & Wilkins customer service representatives are available from 8:30 am to 6 pm, EST.

15 14 13 12 11

For Richard H. Gelberman, MD, our friend, mentor, and colleague, who has inspired us with his passion for education and with his devotion to the field of anatomy.

Contents

Foreword

Knowledge of anatomy is the basic element of successful surgery. John Hunter is recognized as transforming the little regarded practice of surgery in the 18th century to a scientific discipline. He did so in great part by his focus on a detailed understanding of anatomy. His well-organized dissection laboratory, his elegantly prosected specimens, and his lucid lecture presentations established his reputation as a master surgeon and were instrumental in elevating the skills of his students and colleagues.

A Pocketbook Manual of Hand and Upper Extremity Anatomy: Primus Manus will perform a similar role for students of hand surgery in the 21st Century. This well-illustrated and referenced text focuses on the intricate anatomical features of the structures of the hand in great detail and provides appropriate clinical correlations. Doctors Leversedge, Goldfarb, and Boyer have a strong interest in education and their proficiency in teaching is evident in the pages of this text. It is appropriate reading primarily for medical students, residents, fellows, therapists, and clinicians who encounter hand conditions on an occasional basis. Conveniently, the book tucks neatly into a lab coat pocket.

Paul R. Manske

Preface

Hand and upper extremity anatomy forms the basis of a comprehensive understanding of the physiology and pathologic conditions which influence function of the upper limb. Importantly, the intricate relationships and interactions between these diverse tissues define our unique capabilities for human function.

The study of anatomy is analogous to the study of art; one must understand anatomy in order to appreciate it—in order to understand anatomy, however, one must appreciate its complexity of form and function, not withstanding its variations and anomalies.

In an era where time spent in the anatomy laboratory has been de-emphasized within the medical education curriculum, an appreciation for anatomic relationships gained from a hands-on experience may suffer; a lack of awareness for anatomic detail may translate into the unfortunate consequence of a less detailed clinical assessment or a compromised treatment plan.

We embarked on this project with the hope of creating a comprehensive but clinically relevant anatomy reference, from the elbow to the fingertips, which would be portable and readily accessible to all levels of clinical training. As the page limits one to a two-dimensional message, we attempted to create images through our dissections and photography that would portray pertinent relationships from a three-dimensional perspective. We would like to thank our colleagues at Lippincott Williams & Wilkins for their guidance and for their willingness to pursue the project as we envisioned it—particularly, we are grateful to Robert Hurley and Eileen Wolfberg for providing us this opportunity, and the great efforts of Elise Paxson for keeping us moving forward with the production process.

Hopefully, this manual will provide students of hand and upper extremity surgery with an efficient resource for the care of conditions affecting the upper extremity. We are fortunate that our mentors have inspired us to learn and to teach—and there is no topic more pertinent to this mission than to understand and to appreciate the anatomy of the hand and upper extremity, *primus manus*.

Fraser J. Leversedge, MD
Charles A. Goldfarb, MD
Martin I. Boyer, MD

1   Hand

1.1   Osteology and Joints of the Hand

OSTEOLOGY

- Finger: proximal, middle, and distal phalanges
- Thumb: proximal and distal phalanges
- Hand: metacarpals

JOINTS OF THE HAND

Thumb Carpometacarpal (CMC) Joint or Trapeziometacarpal (TM) Joint

- Two reciprocally opposed saddles, orientated 90° to one another
- Architecture permits opposition, circumduction, and prehensile activity
- Bony structure does not provide significant stability
- Joint is stabilized by 16 named ligaments
- Primary stabilizers:
  - **dAOL (anterior oblique or volar beak ligament)** is located opposite to the APL expansion

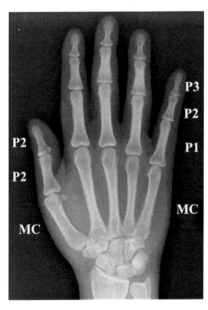

FIGURE 1.1-1 Posteroanterior radiograph of the right hand. MC, metacarpal; P1, proximal phalanx; P2, middle phalanx; P3, distal phalanx.

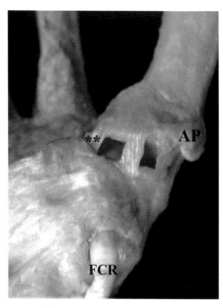

FIGURE 1.1-2 The volar aspect of the thumb carpometacarpal joint (CMC joint). The flexor carpi radialis *(FCR)* tendon angles dorsally at the trapezial groove to insert at the volar base of the index metacarpal. The anterior oblique ligament *(**)* or "volar beak ligament" is the primary stabilizer of the thumb CMC joint. The AOL originates at the beak of the thumb metacarpal base (ulnar volar) and inserts into the volar tubercle of the trapezium. It is taut throughout thumb motion. An insertion of the abductor pollicis longus tendon *(AP)* is the radial base of the thumb metacarpal (cut).

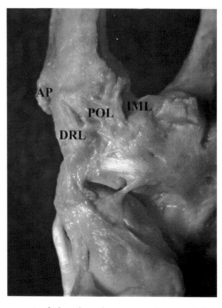

FIGURE 1.1-3 The dorsal aspect of the thumb carpometacarpal joint (CMC joint). The abductor pollicis longus tendon *(AP)* has been cut from its insertion into the radial base of the thumb metacarpal. The dorsoradial ligament *(DRL)* originates at the dorsoradial tubercle of the trapezium and inserts into the dorsal base of the thumb metacarpal. It is taut with thumb adduction and flexion. The posterior oblique ligament *(POL)* runs from the beak of the thumb metacarpal base to the dorsoulnar tubercle of the trapezium. The POL is taut with thumb abduction and flexion. The first intermetacarpal ligament *(IML)* connects the thumb and index metacarpal bases and is taut with thumb abduction.

- **Dorsal ligamentous complex**
  - Posterior oblique ligament (POL)
  - Dorsoradial ligament (DRL)

■ *Clinical Correlate:* During tip and key pinch, approximately 13–14×, the applied force at the thumb tip is measured at the thumb CMC joint.

Metacarpophalangeal (MCP) Joint

Finger

- Condyloid (triaxial) joint
- Typical range of motion: 15° hyperextension to 90° flexion
- **CAM effect** for collateral ligaments due to shape of metacarpal head. The collateral ligaments taut with MCP joint flexion/lax in extension.
- MCP joint stable in flexion (vs. extension) due to trapezoidal shape of metacarpal head and ligamentous laxity in extension.

■ *Clinical Correlate:* To keep the collateral ligaments from shortening, the MCP joint should be immobilized in flexion.

Thumb

- Metacarpal head is a single, broad condyle. It is rounded in 90% of people and is flat in 10%.
- Sesamoids are contained within the substance of the volar plate
- Radial sesamoid is larger and is a **site of FPB insertion**
- Wide variation in "normal" range of motion
- Ulnar collateral ligament (UCL) includes proper and accessory portions
  - Stability of the UCL should be tested with the MCP joint in full extension and in 30° flexion
  - UCL tensile strength ~36 kg

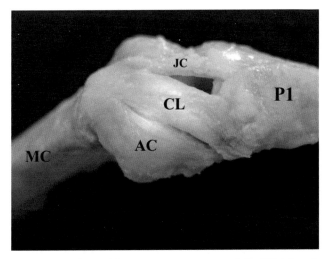

FIGURE 1.1-4 Similar to the collateral ligament arrangement of the PIP joint, the metacarpophalangeal joint (MCP joint) collateral ligament includes a proper collateral ligament *(CL)* and an accessory collateral ligament *(AC)*. Both take their origin at the dorsal-lateral aspect of the head of the metacarpal; the CL inserts into the lateral base of the proximal phalanx *(P1)* and the AC inserts into the volar plate. There is a more developed joint capsule *(JC)* than appreciated at the PIP joint.

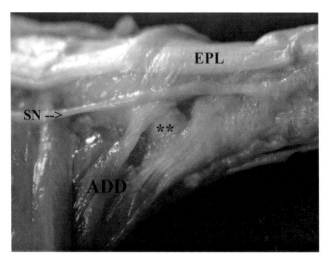

FIGURE 1.1-5 The ulnar aspect of the thumb metacarpophalangeal joint (MCP joint) is exposed, demonstrating the insertion of the adductor aponeurosis *(ADD)* into the dorsal apparatus (stabilizing retinaculum of the extensor pollicis longus tendon *(EPL)*), the ulnar sesamoid of the thumb, and the ulnar base of the proximal phalanx. Often, there are multiple sensory nerve branches *(SN)* traversing the ulnar margin of the MCP joint region. The ulnar collateral ligament of the thumb MCP joint is identified deep to the adductor aponeurosis *(**)*.

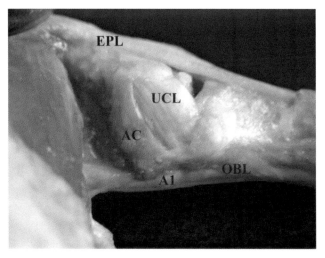

FIGURE 1.1-6 The adductor aponeurosis has been removed (from Figure 1.1-5), revealing the ulnar aspect of the thumb metacarpophalangeal joint (MCP joint). The ulnar collateral ligament *(UCL)* and the accessory ulnar collateral ligament *(AC)* originate at the dorsal ulnar margin of the head of the metacarpal; the UCL inserts into the ulnar base of the proximal phalanx and the AC inserts into the volar plate of the MCP joint. The extensor pollicis longus tendon *(EPL)* is dorsal to the MP joint and the A1 and oblique *(OBL)* pulleys of the flexor sheath are noted volar to the MP joint and the proximal phalanx.

■ *Clinical Correlate:* A **Stener lesion** occurs when UCL is torn from its insertion on base of proximal phalanx and is trapped proximal to adductor pollicis aponeurosis. The adductor aponeurosis prevents the ligament from returning to its native position and thus prevents healing.

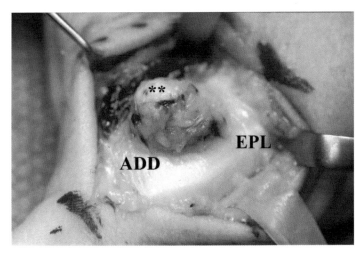

FIGURE 1.1-7 Intra-operative photograph of a Stener lesion involving the avulsion of the UCL insertion such that it is trapped proximal and superficial to the adductor aponeurosis (ADD). EPL, extensor pollicis longus tendon.

Proximal Interphalangeal (PIP) Joint

- A hinge joint
- Head of proximal phalanx includes two condyles separated by an **intercondylar notch** that provides some inherent joint stability through its articulation with the **median ridge** at the base of the middle phalanx.
- Collateral ligaments are taut throughout range of motion; therefore, there is no CAM effect as observed in the MCP joint.
- **Proper collateral ligament**: origin at pit on head of proximal phalanx; insertion at lateral tubercle of middle phalanx base.
- **Accessory collateral ligament**: inserts into volar plate and provides greater joint stability in extension.
- The **volar plate** is a thick, fibrocartilagenous floor that originates deep to the A2 pulley and inserts into the "rough area" at the base of P2; it supports the insertion of the accessory collateral ligament and prevents PIP joint hyperextension.
- At the base of the middle phalanx:
  - **Dorsal tubercle**—insertion of central slip
  - **Lateral tubercle**—insertion of collateral ligaments
  - Volar insertions from proximal to distal:
    - Volar plate
    - FDS tendon
    - A4 pulley
- The **"check" ligaments** are the reflected fibers of the flexor sheath/lateral margin of the volar plate.

■ *Clinical Correlate:* The "checkrein ligament" involves the pathologic thickening of the check ligaments that contribute to a PIP joint flexion contracture.

Distal Interphalangeal (DIP) Joint

- Stabilized by the collateral ligaments, the terminal extensor tendon insertion, the FDP insertion, and the volar plate.

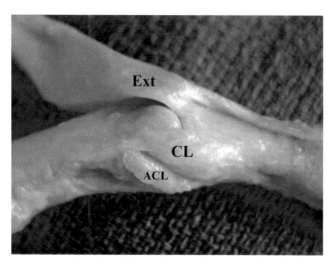

FIGURE 1.1-8 Lateral view of the proximal interphalangeal joint (PIP joint). The central slip of the extensor tendon *(Ext)* inserts into the dorsal tubercle of the base of the middle phalanx. The proper collateral ligament *(CL)* takes its origin at the lateral aspect of the head of the proximal phalanx and inserts into the lateral tubercle of the base of the middle phalanx. The accessory collateral ligament *(ACL)*, which is taut in PIP joint extension, inserts into the volar plate of the PIP joint.

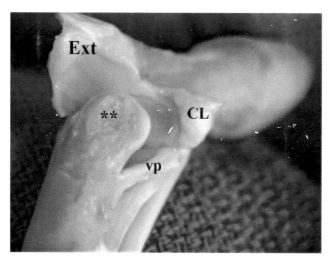

FIGURE 1.1-9 An oblique view of the PIP joint with the collateral ligament *(CL)* reflected from its origin at the head of the proximal phalanx reveals the "pit" at the lateral aspect of the head of the proximal phalanx *(**)*. The volar plate *(vp)* strongly resists PIP joint hyperextension and supports the insertion of the accessory collateral ligament (Figure 1). The central slip *(Ext)* is elevated at its insertion into the dorsal tubercle of the middle phalanx.

RECOMMENDED READING

Bailie DS, Benson LS, Marymount JV. Proximal interphalangeal joint injuries of the hand, part I: anatomy and diagnosis. *Am J Orthop*. 1996;25:474–477.

Barmakian JT. Anatomy of the joints of the thumb. *Hand Clin*. 1992;8:683–691.

Bettinger PC, Linscheid RL, Berger RA, et al. An anatomic study of the stabilizing ligaments of the trapezium and trapeziometacarpal joint. *J Hand Surg*. 1999;24A:786–798.

Heyman P, Gelberman RH, Duncan K, et al. Injuries of the ulnar collateral ligament of the thumb metacarpophalangeal joint. Biomechanical and prospective clinical studies on the usefulness of valgus stress testing. *Clin Orthop Relat Res*. 1993;292:165–171.

Kuczynski K. Carpometacarpal joint of the human thumb. *J Anat.* 1974;118:119.

Kuczynski K. The proximal interphalangeal joint. Anatomy and causes of stiffness in the fingers. *J Bone Joint Surg.* 1968;50B:656–663.

Leibovic SJ, Bowers WH. Anatomy of the proximal interphalangeal joint. *Hand Clin.* 1994;10:169–178.

Leversedge FJ. Anatomy and pathomechanics of the thumb. *Hand Clin.* 2008;24:219–229.

Pellegrini VD Jr. Osteoarthritis of the trapeziometacarpal joint: the pathophysiology of articular cartilage degeneration. I. Anatomy and pathology of the aging joint. *J Bone Joint Surg.* 1991;16A:967–974.

Stener B. Displacement of the ruptured ulnar collateral ligament of the metacarpophalangeal joint of the thumb. A clinical and anatomical study. *J Bone Joint Surg.* 1962;44B:869–879.

1.2   Nail Bed

- **Perionychium**—Entire area of the nail, nail bed, and surrounding skin.
- **Paronychium**—Lateral nail fold; soft tissue/skin directly surrounding the nail.
- **Hyponychium**—Skin immediately distal and palmar to the nail, at the junction of the sterile matrix and fingertip skin. Sensate and protective against infection.
- **Eponychium**—Dorsal nail fold, proximal to nail plate. Adds shine to nail.
- **Lunula**—White portion of proximal nail. Color is most likely due to retained cell nuclei during growth process.
- **Sterile matrix**—Soft tissue deep and adherent to the nail, distal to lunula. Contributes to the thickening of the nail.
- **Germinal matrix**—Soft tissue deep to the nail and proximal to the sterile matrix (includes lunula). Responsible for majority of nail development.
- **Periosteum** of the distal phalanx is immediately volar to the sterile and germinal matrices.
- **Extensor tendon insertion (terminal tendon)**—Average distance to proximal germinal matrix approximately 1.2 to 1.4 mm.

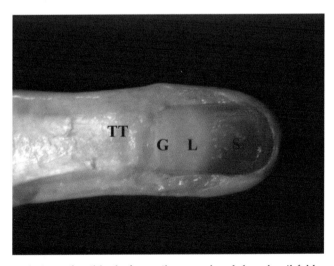

FIGURE 1.2-1 Dorsal view of nail bed after nail removal and dorsal nail fold removal demonstrating the terminal extensor tendon *(TT)*, germinal matrix *(G)*, lunula *(L)*, and sterile matrix *(S)*.

■ *Clinical Correlate:* Paronychia—Infection involving the area of the paronychium, which usually develops along lateral nail fold and may spread to eponychium. While the condition may begin with cellulitis alone, surgical treatment is required to drain abscess.

■ *Clinical Correlate:* Nail bed injury—Crush injury or distal phalanx fracture may lead to disruption of germinal or sterile matrix. Anatomical repair provides highest likelihood of normal nail growth. The dorsal nail fold is splinted away from underlying germinal matrix to prevent scarring that may otherwise limit nail growth.

RECOMMENDED READING

Schweitzer TP, Rayan GM. The terminal tendon of the digital extensor mechanism, part I: anatomic study. *J Hand Surg.* 2004;29A:898–902.
Shum C, Bruno RJ, Ristic S, et al. Examination of the anatomic relationship of the proximal germinal matrix to the extensor tendon insertion. *J Hand Surg.* 2000;25A:1114–1117.
Zook EG. Anatomy and physiology of the perionychium. *Hand Clin.* 2002;18(4):553–559.
Zook EG, Van Beek AL, Russell RC, et al. Anatomy and physiology of the perionychium: a review of the literature and anatomical study. *J Hand Surg.* 1980;5:528–536.

1.3   Dorsal Digit

DORSAL APPARATUS (Figs. 1.3-2 to 1.3-4)

• Extensor tendons are divided into anatomic zones

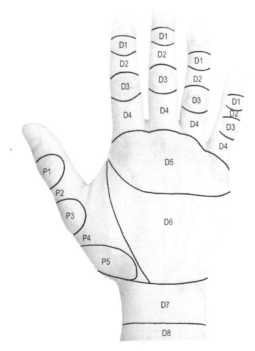

FIGURE 1.3-1 Illustration describing the zones of extensor tendon injuries.

- The extrinsic extensor tendon trifurcates at the base of P1 with the central portion inserting into the dorsal base of P2 as the **central slip**.
- The lateral slips are joined by contributions from the **oblique fibers** of the lumbricals to form the **conjoined lateral band**.
- The conjoined lateral bands converge over the middle phalanx to form the **terminal tendon** that inserts into the dorsal base of the distal phalanx where it functions to extend the DIP joint.
- Interosseous and lumbrical contributions to dorsal apparatus:

Interosseous Muscles:

- Four dorsal (abductors) and three volar (adductors)
- All tendons pass **dorsal to the deep transverse intermetacarpal ligament** (in contrast to lumbricals and neurovascular bundles that pass volar to the ligament)

Dorsal Interosseous:

- Bipennate (arise from both adjacent metacarpals)
- In general, innervated by the ulnar nerve
- Abduct the digit away from the central axis of the hand (long finger ray)
- Located on the radial side of the index and long; ulnar side of the long and ring fingers
- The index dorsal interosseous (DI) inserts solely through the medial tendon into the base of the proximal phalanx making it a strong abductor. The other dorsal interossei

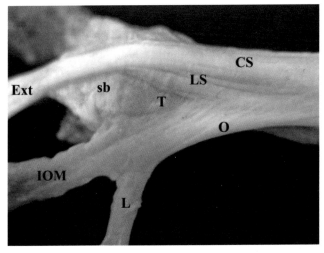

FIGURE 1.3-2 The dorsal digital extensor apparatus is derived from contributions of the extrinsic extensor tendons and the intrinsic musculature of the hand. The extrinsic extensor tendon *(Ext)* is identified at the level of the distal hand and splits into two lateral slips *(LS)* and the central tendon slip *(CS)*. At the dorsal MCP joint, the extensor tendon is stabilized by the vertically orientated fibers of the sagittal band *(sb)*, which originate from the radial and ulnar sides of the volar plate of the MCP joint and the volar base of the proximal phalanx. The MCP joint is extended via a sling-like mechanism of the sagittal band as there is no direct fiber insertion from the extrinsic extensor tendon at the proximal phalanx. The deep head of the interosseous muscle *(IOM)* courses superficial to the sagittal band *(sb)* at the level of the MP joint and runs parallel and distal to the sagittal band over the proximal phalanx to form the transverse fibers *(T)* of the extensor apparatus. The lumbrical muscle *(L)* on the radial aspect of the digit forms the oblique fibers *(O)* of the extensor apparatus, which join with the lateral slip of the extrinsic extensor tendon to form the conjoined lateral band *(CLB)*.

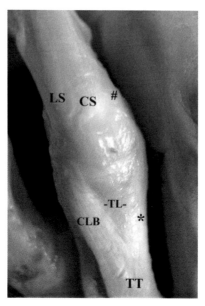

FIGURE 1.3-3 The extrinsic extensor tendon divides into a central slip *(CS)* and two lateral slips (LS and #). The central slip inserts at the dorsal base of the middle phalanx to extend the PIP joint and the two lateral slips receive contributory fibers from the lumbricals via oblique fibers of the extensor hood to form the conjoined lateral bands (**CLB** and *). These conjoined lateral bands coalesce to form the terminal tendon *(TT)* that inserts at the dorsal base of the distal phalanx to extend the DIP joint. The triangular ligament *(TL)* stabilizes the conjoined lateral bands from volar subluxation.

insert in mixed fashion into the proximal phalanx and the transverse fibers to both abduct and flex the MCP joint.
- The small finger abductor is the **abductor digiti minimi**.
- **Superficial muscle belly**—travels **deep to sagittal band** as the medial tendon to insert into the lateral tubercle of P1.
- **Deep muscle belly**—travels **superficial to the sagittal band** as the lateral tendon to become the **transverse fibers of the lateral band**, which flex the MP joint. The transverse fibers run parallel to the sagittal band but are more distal over the proximal phalanx.
- **Insertions**
  - **1st DI**—100% medial tendon
  - **2nd DI**—60% medial tendon + 40% lateral tendon
  - **3rd DI**—6% medial tendon + 94% lateral tendon
  - **4th DI**—40% medial tendon + 60% lateral tendon

Volar Interosseous:
- Unipennate
- In general, innervated by the ulnar nerve
- Adduct and flex P1
- No insertion on P1; insertion into lateral band on adductor side of index, ring, and small fingers

Transverse Fibers:
- Approximate the level of the mid-third P1
- Arch dorsally from lateral tendon on intrinsic apparatus to surround the trifurcating extensor tendon

- Runs in similar orientation to sagittal bands; sagittal bands are part of extrinsic apparatus and transverse fibers are part of intrinsic apparatus
- Serve as insertion of interossei that facilitate MCP joint flexion

■ *Clinical Correlate:* **Intrinsic tightness** may occur following trauma and scarring of the interossei muscle. Testing is positive when it is difficult to passively flex the PIP joint with the MCP joint held in extension, but easier to passively flex the PIP joint when the MCP joint is held in flexion.

Lumbrical Muscles:

- Origin: FDP tendon in palm.
- Tendons pass **volar to the deep intermetacarpal ligament** with neurovascular bundles and radial to MCP joint.
- Insert on the radial side of each digit through the **oblique fibers of the intrinsic apparatus**.
- Fibers join the lateral slip (from extrinsic extensor tendon) to form the **conjoined lateral band**.
- Contribute to PIP joint extension (through direct insertion at base of P2) and DIP joint extension (through conjoined lateral bands/terminal tendon insertion).
- The two radial-most lumbrical muscles are innervated by motor branches of the common digital nerves from the median nerve and are typically **unipennate**.
- The two ulnar-most muscles are innervated by motor branches off of the deep branch of the ulnar nerve directly and are typically **bipennate**.
- The lumbricals are unique in that they can relax their antagonist muscle (FDP).

Oblique Fibers:

- Insert into dorsolateral tubercles of P2 through the medial bands
- Assists central slip with PIP extension
- Insert—with lateral slips of extrinsic apparatus—into conjoined lateral bands through the lateral bands
- Assists with DIP extension

■ *Clinical Correlate:* A **lumbrical-plus finger** involves the paradoxical extension of the interphalangeal joints as a patient attempts to actively flex the finger. This occurs when the FDP motor unit is activated, but fails to act on the DIP joint due to a loss of relative FDP tendon excursion distal to the lumbrical origin secondary to FDP injury (i.e., laceration, avulsion, and peritendinous adhesions). The proximal FDP motor unit then acts through the intact lumbrical, causing extension of the interphalangeal joints.

Motor unit	Action via	Action
Extensor tendon	Sagittal band	MCP joint extension
Interosseous	Transverse fibers	MCP joint flexion
Lumbrical	Oblique fibers	PIP joint extension

DORSAL STABILIZING STRUCTURES

Sagittal Bands

- Continuation of the dorsal intertendinous fascia
- Originate on both sides of the MCP joint, from the lateral margins of the volar plate and volar periosteum of the base of the proximal phalanx
- Typically are 15 to 20 mm in length

- Functions:
  - Contribute indirectly to MCP joint extension through sling-like mechanism. There is usually no direct bony insertion of the extrinsic extensors at the dorsal base of the proximal phalanx.
  - Prevent extensor tendon bowstringing
  - Stabilize the extrinsic extensor tendon centrally, over the dorsal aspect of the MCP joint
  - Limit extensor digitorum communis (EDC) excursion
  - Contribute indirectly to MCP joint's lateral stability in MCP extension
- Medial tendon of the interosseous m. passes deep to the sagittal band to insert on the lateral tubercle of P1 (abduction)
- Lateral tendon of the interosseous m. passes superficial to the sagittal band to insert into the transverse fibers of the dorsal apparatus (MCP joint flexion)

■ *Clinical Correlate:* Injury to the sagittal band may result in subluxation of the extrinsic extensor tendons.

Triangular Ligament (Fig. 1.3-3)

- Connects the conjoined lateral bands over the dorsal aspect of the middle phalanx to prevent volar subluxation of conjoined lateral bands with flexion
- Base: central slip attachment
- Sides: conjoined lateral bands
- Apex: terminal tendon

■ *Clinical Correlate:* Injury to the triangular ligament allows the conjoined lateral bands to subluxate volarly and may contribute to the formation of a flexion contracture of the PIP joint and/or a boutonnière deformity.

Transverse Retinacular Ligament (Fig. 1.3-4)

- Fibers are orientated in dorsal–volar direction at level of PIP joint
- Prevents dorsal subluxation of the conjoined lateral bands

■ *Clinical Correlate:* Injury to the transverse retinacular ligament allows the conjoined lateral bands to subluxate dorsally and may contribute to an extended or hyperextended posture of the PIP joint and an associated swan-neck deformity.

Oblique Retinacular Ligament (ORL)—of Landsmeer (Fig. 1.3-4)

- Serves to link composite flexion and extension of PIP and DIP joints
  - With PIP in extension, ORL tightens and thus extends DIP joint
  - When DIP flexes, ORL tightens and PIP flexes also
- Originates at fibro-osseous gutter at the A2 pulley and middle 1/3 proximal phalanx and runs distally to insert into the terminal extensor tendon dorsally
- The ORL lies volar to the PIP joint and dorsal to the DIP joint
- Active PIP joint flexion results in decreased ORL tension, allowing for active DIP joint flexion
- Schrewsbury
  - ORL present in only 40% to 50% of cadaver dissection, except ulnar side of ring finger (~90%)

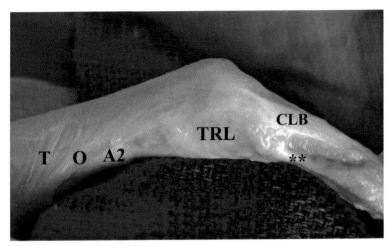

FIGURE 1.3-4 The extensor hood is made up of contributions from tendons of the deep head of the interosseous muscles as the transverse fibers *(T)* and from the lumbrical tendons as the oblique fibers *(O)*. The deep head of the interosseous muscle courses superficial to the sagittal band at the level of the MCP joint and run parallel and distal to the sagittal band over the proximal phalanx. The transverse fibers of the extensor apparatus flex the MP joint. The oblique fibers of the dorsal apparatus join the lateral slip of the extrinsic extensor tendon to form the conjoined lateral band *(CLB)*. These fibers contribute to PIP joint extension and to DIP joint extension (via the terminal tendon). The CLB is stabilized from dorsal translation by the transverse retinacular ligament *(TRL)*; the TRL fibers run in a volar–dorsal orientation from the flexor sheath to the lateral margin of the CLB. The oblique retinacular ligament *(ORL)* passively links the PIP and DIP joints as it travels from volar to dorsal from the fibro-osseous gutter (middle 1/3 of the proximal phalanx and A2 pulley *(A2)*) to the proximal aspect of the distal phalanx through the extensor tendon.

■ *Clinical Correlate:* ORL reconstruction can help reestablish the link between the PIP and DIP joints. Clinically, this surgery may be helpful for the treatment of a chronic mallet finger combined with secondary hyperextension of the PIP joint.

Dorsal Thumb

- At the MCP joint, the EPL tendon is ulnar to the EPB tendon before flattening and continuing to its insertion at the dorsal base of the distal phalanx.
- The EPL and EPB are stabilized by the sagittal band at the MCP joint and are connected by retinaculum.
- Variable EPB anatomy has been described, including its insertion into the extensor hood without its typical insertion into the proximal phalanx.
- The thumb ulnar and radial components of the sagittal band arise from a soft tissue confluence at the volar MCP joint and insert onto their respective margins of the EPL tendon. Deficit of the radial sagittal band results in EPL instability.

RECOMMENDED READING

al-Qattan MM, Robertson GA. An anatomical study of the deep transverse metacarpal ligament. *J Anat.* 1993;182:443–446.

Boyer MI, Gelberman RH. Operative correction of swan-neck and boutonniere deformities in the rheumatoid hand. *J Am Acad Orthop Surg.* 1999;7:92–100.

Brunelli GA, Brunelli GR. Anatomy of the extensor pollicis brevis muscle. *J Hand Surg.* 1992;17B:267–269.

Doyle JR, Blythe WF. Anatomy of the flexor tendon sheath and pulleys of the thumb. *J Hand Surg.* 1977;2A:149–151.

Harris C, Rutledge GL. The functional anatomy of the extensor mechanism of the finger. *J Bone Joint Surg.* 1972;54A:713–726.

Jaibaji M, Rayan GM, Chung KW. Functional anatomy of the thumb sagittal band. *J Hand Surg.* 2008;33A:879–884.

Kanaya K, Wada T, Isogai S, et al. Variation in insertion of the abductor digiti minimi: an anatomic study. *J Hand Surg.* 2002;27A:325–328.

Landsmeer JM. The anatomy of the dorsal aponeurosis of the human finger and its functional significance. *Anat Rec.* 1949;104:31–44.

Littler JW. The finger extensor mechanism. *Surg Clin North Am.* 1967;47:415–432.

Schweitzer TP, Rayan GM. The terminal tendon of the digital extensor mechanism, part I: anatomic study. *J Hand Surg.* 2004;29A:898–902.

Schrewsbury MM, Johnson RK. A systematic study of the oblique retinacular ligament of the human finger: its structure and function. *J Hand Surg.* 1977;2A:194–199.

Smith RJ. Intrinsic muscles of the fingers: function, dysfunction, and surgical reconstruction. In: *AAOS Instructional Course Lecture*, vol. 24. St. Louis, MO: C. V. Mosby; 1975:200–220.

Tubiana R, Valentin P. Anatomy of the extensor apparatus of the fingers. *Surg Clin North Am.* 1964;44:897–906.

Tubiana R, Valentin P. The physiology of the extension of the fingers. *Surg Clin North Am.* 1964;44:907–918.

von Schroeder HP, Botte MJ. Functional anatomy of the extensor tendons of the digits. *Hand Clin.* 1997;13:51–62.

Young CM, Rayan GM. The sagittal band: anatomic and biomechanical study. *J Hand Surg.* 2000;25A:1107–1113.

1.4   Palmar Hand and Digit

PALMAR FASCIA

- Palmar aponeurosis
  - Palmaris longus terminates into the palmar fascia/aponeurosis
- Pretendinous band
  - Longitudinal fascial bands of the palm
  - Superficial to the transverse fibers of palmar aponeurosis (ligament of Skoog)
  - Inserts into skin at level of MCP joint
  - Trifurcates into spiral bands (radial + ulnar) and central band
- Superficial transverse metacarpal ligament
  - Transverse fibers of palmar aponeurosis (ligament of Skoog)
- Natatory ligament
  - Transverse fibers at the palmodigital crease; restrict digital abduction
- Vertical septa of Legeau and Juvara
  - Vertical septa (8) on each side of flexor tendons to create seven longitudinal compartments; four containing flexor tendons and three containing neurovascular bundles and lumbricals.
  - Septa attached to the transverse ligament of palmar aponeurosis (superficial) and to the interpalmar plate ligament (deep).
- Deep transverse intermetacarpal ligament or interpalmar plate ligament
  - Lumbricals and neurovascular bundles pass superficial to the deep transverse intermetacarpal ligament; the interossei travel dorsal to the ligament.

■ *Clinical Correlate:* **Dupuytren's disease** affects the longitudinal fibers of the palmar aponeurosis and may lead to contractures of the MCP and PIP joints. Transverse and vertical fascia (i.e., superficial and deep transverse intermetacarpal ligaments and septa of Legeau and Juvara) are typically spared in Dupuytren disease.

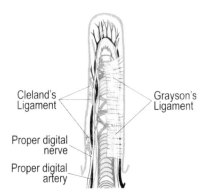

FIGURE 1.4-1 Illustration of the palmar finger, demonstrating the contributions of Grayson's ligament and Cleland's ligament to the lateral digital sheath. Grayson's ligament originates from the volar flexor sheath, its fibers running perpendicular to the longitudinal axis of the digit, to insert into the skin. Grayson's ligament is volar or palmar to the digital neurovascular bundle. Cleland's ligament involves two ligaments arising obliquely from each side of the DIP joint, and two ligaments arising obliquely from each side of the PIP joint; the ligaments are dorsal to the digital neurovascular bundles and originate from the phalanx and insert into the skin.

DIGITAL FASCIA

- Lateral digital sheet (Fig. 1.4-1)—receives contributions from:
  1. Spiral band
     - Originates at pretendinous band; pass dorsal to n-v bundle to insert on lateral digital sheet
  2. Natatory ligament
     - Transverse fibers at the palmodigital crease
  3. Grayson's ligaments
     - Arise from volar aspect of flexor tendon sheath and insert into skin
     - Volar to digital neurovascular bundles
     - Fibers orientated perpendicular to longitudinal digital axis
  4. Cleland's ligaments
     - Fibers originate from the phalanges, diverge, and insert into skin
     - Four ligaments on each side of finger; two adjacent to PIP joint and two adjacent to DIP joint
     - Dorsal to digital neurovascular bundles
     - PIP bundles (two sets) and DIP bundles (two sets)
- Grayson's and Cleland's ligaments serve to anchor the skin during digital motion and to stabilize the digital neurovascular bundles during digital flexion.

FLEXOR TENDON—FINGER

- Flexor tendons are divided into **five anatomic zones**
- FDS enters flexor sheath volar to FDP
- At the level of the A1 pulley, the FDS flattens and bifurcates to allow the deeper FDP to pass distally to its insertion at the base of the distal phalanx.
- The bifurcating limbs of FDS rotate laterally and dorsally around FDP and then divide again into medial and lateral slips. **Medial slips** cross dorsal to FDP, rejoining (**chiasma tendinum of Camper**) over the distal aspect of the proximal phalanx and PIP joint volar plate. The **lateral slips** continue distally to insert at base of the middle phalanx.
- FDP continues distally to insert into volar base of distal phalanx.

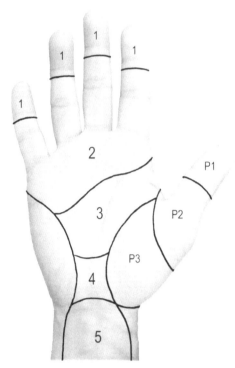

FIGURE 1.4-2 Anatomical zones for the characterization of flexor tendon injuries.

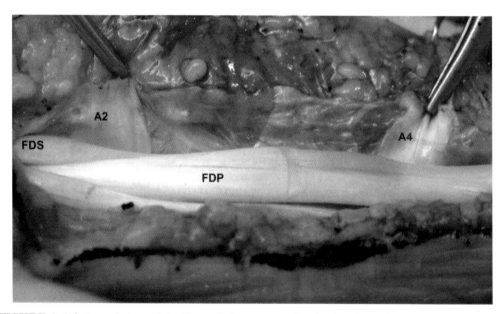

FIGURE 1.4-3 Lateral view of the flexor digitorum superficialis *(FDS)* and flexor digitorum profundus *(FDP)* tendons within the digit. The flexor sheath has been elevated *(forceps)* demonstrating the improved definition of the flexor pulleys from within the flexor sheath. The *(A2)* and *(A4)* pulleys are labeled; the A3 pulley that overlays the PIP joint is a slightly less dense and thinner region of the sheath between the A2 and A4 pulleys. Oblique fibers of the cruciate pulleys are seen in the membranous portion of the flexor sheath, between the annular pulleys. The FDP tendon emerges from its dorsal position, coursing between the inserting slips of the FDS tendon to continue distally along the digit.

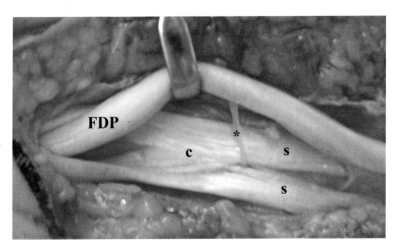

FIGURE 1.4-4 The bifurcating limbs of the FDS tendon rotate laterally and dorsally around the **FDP** tendon and then divide again into medial and lateral slips. The medial slips cross dorsal to the FDP tendon, rejoining as the chiasma tendinum of Camper *(c)* over the distal aspect of the proximal phalanx and PIP joint volar plate. The lateral slip *(s)* continues distally to insert at the volar base of the middle phalanx. The vinculum longum to the profundus tendon *(*)* is identified as it penetrates the FDS from dorsal to volar.

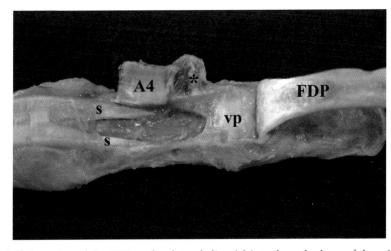

FIGURE 1.4-5 Insertion of the FDS tendon lateral slips *(s)* into the volar base of the middle phalanx at the level of the A4 pulley (reflected). The A5 pulley is identified *(*)*. The FDP tendon has been reflected distally, revealing the swallowtail origin and substance of the DIP joint volar plate *(vp)*.

- Dual source of flexor tendon nutrition:
  1. **Direct vascular** (Figs. 1.4-6 and 1.4-7)
     - Transverse digital arteries ("ladder branches") arise from digital arteries to supply the vincular system. The vincula tendina are mesotendinous vascular networks on the dorsal surface of the flexor tendons.
       - Proximal transverse digital artery—origin between A2 and A3 pulleys; supplies VBS + VLP
       - Interphalangeal transverse digital artery—origin between A3 and A4 pulleys; supplies VBP
       - Distal transverse digital artery—origin between A4 and A5 pulleys; supplies VBP

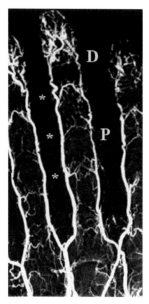

FIGURE 1.4-6 Arterial perfusion of the long finger demonstrating the transversely oriented "ladder" branches arising from the digital arteries (*). The proximal interphalangeal *(P)* and distal interphalangeal *(D)* joints are noted for reference.

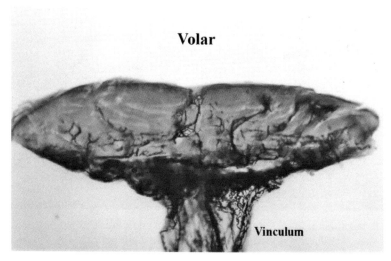

FIGURE 1.4-7 Transverse section of the intrasynovial portion of the digital flexor tendon (clarified following India ink arterial injection) demonstrating the dorsal vincula or mesotenon. The vincula arises from the digital arterial "ladder" branches and contributes to the nutritional supply of the dorsal flexor tendon.

- Vinculum longum superficialis (VLS)—at base of proximal phalanx
- Vinculum breve superficialis (VBS)—at volar plate of PIP joint
- Vinculum longum profundus (VLP)—variable origin
- Vinculum breve profundus (VBP)—at distal aspect of middle phalanx
- Direct arterial supply from intraosseous vessels at tendinous insertions
2. Synovial diffusion
   - Avascular/hypovascular zones of FDS and FDP within the flexor sheath rely on intratendinous cannaliculi for synovial diffusion.

■ *Clinical Correlate:* Independent active flexion of the small finger PIP joint may be absent due to variability in the development of the FDS to the small finger (hypoplastic or absent).

■ *Clinical Correlate:* The "**quadrigia effect**" reflects a lack of independent active motion of the FDP tendons due to their common muscular origin (index FDP independence may vary). If the tension of one FDP muscle-tendon unit is altered (i.e., overadvancement during repair and relative tendon shortening or an overlengthening of a tendon graft), the functioning of the other FDP tendons is affected. Therefore, if the FDP is relatively shortened during advancement/repair, the affected digit will have the potential to flex fully, while the other digits will lack full flexion due to their relative "lengthening" compared to the repaired tendon.

FLEXOR SHEATH/PULLEYS (Figs. 1.4-8 and 1.4-9)

- Fibro-osseous digital sheath provides both biomechanical efficiency and a source of nutrition to the flexor tendons.
- The flexor sheath to the index, long, and ring fingers runs from the metacarpal neck to the DIP joint.
- The small finger flexor sheath may connect with the ulnar bursa, proximally.
- Flexor tendons are enveloped by a layer of **visceral paratenon**.
- Pulley/retinacular system is lined by a layer of **parietal paratenon**.
- Condensations of the synovial sheath, or flexor pulleys, form at strategic points along the digit to work in conjunction with the transverse carpal ligament and the palmar aponeurosis pulley to maximize efficiency of joint rotation and force transmission.
- Five annular and three cruciform pulleys are typically described:

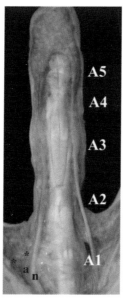

FIGURE 1.4-8 Palmar finger dissection with the digital flexor sheath intact. Condensations of the flexor sheath form annular and cruciate pulleys that maximize the biomechanical efficiency of the flexor apparatus. The annular pulleys *(A1–A5)* are identified along the right side of the digit. The common digital nerves divide into their respective radial and ulnar proper digital nerves in the distal palm, typically proximal to the division of the common digital arteries into their associated proper digital arteries *(*)*. In the distal palm, the digital nerve *(n)* lies palmar to the digital artery *(a)*.

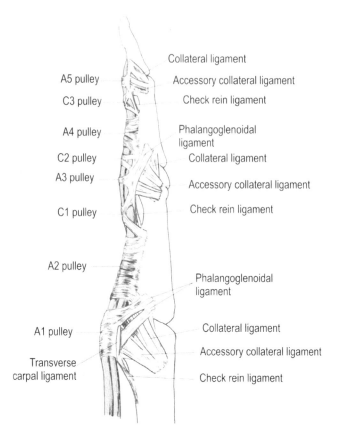

A5 pulley
C3 pulley

A4 pulley

C2 pulley
A3 pulley

C1 pulley

A2 pulley

A1 pulley

Transverse
carpal ligament

Collateral ligament
Accessory collateral ligament
Check rein ligament

Phalangoglenoidal
ligament
Collateral ligament

Accessory collateral ligament

Check rein ligament

Phalangoglenoidal
ligament

Collateral ligament

Accessory collateral ligament

Check rein ligament

FIGURE 1.4-9 Illustration of the flexor sheath and digital pulley system of the finger.

Annular Pulleys

- A1, A3, A5 pulleys take their origin from palmar plates of the MCP, PIP, and DIP joints, respectively.
- A2 and A4 pulleys originate from the proximal and middle phalanges, respectively.
- A2 is 17 mm in length (longest pulley).
- **A2 and A4 pulleys** are the strongest and most important pulleys, biomechanically; tendon excursion required for full active digital and wrist flexion is minimally increased as long as A2 + A4 pulleys are intact.

Cruciate Pulleys

- Less substantial; located between the annular pulleys
  - C1—between A2 and A3
  - C2—between A3 and A4
  - C3—between A4 and A5
- Palmar aponeurosis pulley is proximal to the A1 pulley and is approximately 9 mm in length. Its importance is increased if other pulleys are absent.

■ *Clinical Correlate:* Classic signs of a flexor sheath infection (**Kanavel's signs**) include: (i) flexed posture of digit; (ii) fusiform swelling of digit, or "sausage digit"; (iii) pain with passive digital extension; and (iv) pain with palpation along the volar digit.

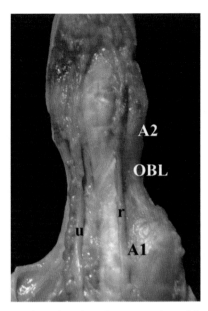

FIGURE 1.4-10 The volar aspect of the thumb with preservation of the digital flexor sheath. The transverse orientation of the A1 and A2 pulleys are identified at the level of the MCP joint and the distal aspect of the proximal phalanx, respectively. The oblique pulley *(OBL)* fibers are orientated from proximal-ulnar to distal-radial. Note the proximity of the radial *(r)* ≫ ulnar *(u)* digital nerve to the A1 pulley.

FLEXOR TENDON—THUMB

- The flexor pollicis longus (FPL) emerges from the interval between the adductor muscle and the FPB/opponens muscles to enter the fibro-osseous digital sheath at the level of the MCP joint.
- The FPL flexes the thumb interphalangeal joint.

FLEXOR SHEATH/PULLEYS—THUMB

- The thumb flexor sheath runs from the wrist crease to the interphalangeal joint.
- The **A1, oblique, and A2 pulleys** comprise the pulley system of the thumb.
- The A1 pulley is at the level of the MCP joint.
- Oblique pulley fibers are orientated in a **distal and radial direction** at the level of the proximal phalanx.
- The A2 pulley originates from the interphalangeal joint volar plate.
- **The A1 and oblique pulleys** are most important, biomechanically.

■ *Clinical Correlate:* The **radial digital nerve** is at particular risk during A1 pulley release due to its oblique course, its proximity to the A1 pulley, and its direct subcutaneous position.

RECOMMENDED READING

Austin GJ, Leslie BM, Ruby LK. Variations of the flexor digitorum superficialis of the small finger. *J Hand Surg.* 1989;14A:262–267.

Bayat A, Shaaban H, Glakas G, et al. The pulley system of the thumb: anatomic and biomechanical study. *J Hand Surg.* 2002;27A:628–635.

Bilderback KK, Rayan GM. The septa of Legeau and Juvara: an anatomic study. *J Hand Surg.* 2004;29:494–499.

Doyle JR. Anatomy of the flexor tendon sheath and pulley system. *J Hand Surg.* 1988;13:473–484.

Doyle JR, Blythe WF. Anatomy of the flexor tendon sheath and pulleys of the thumb. *J Hand Surg.* 1977;2:149–151.

Idler RS. Anatomy and biomechanics of the digital flexor tendons. *Hand Clin.* 1985;1:3–11.

Leversedge FJ, Ditsios K, Goldfarb CA, et al. Vascular anatomy of the human flexor digitorum profundus tendon insertion. *J Hand Surg.* 2002;27A:806–812.

Lin GT, Cooney WP, Amadio PC, et al. Mechanical properties of human pulleys. *J Hand Surg.* 1990;15B:429–434.

Lundborg G, Myrhage R. The vascularization and structure of the human digital tendon sheath as related to flexor tendon function. An angiographic and histological study. *J Hand Surg.* 1977;2:417–427.

Manske PR, Lesker PA. Palmar aponeurosis pulley. *J Hand Surg.* 1983;8:259–263.

McFarlane RM. Patterns of disease fascia in the fingers in Dupuytren's contracture. *Plast Reconstr Surg.* 1974;54:31–44.

Netscher D, Lee M, Thornby J, et al. The effect of division of the transverse carpal ligament on flexor tendon excursion. *J Hand Surg.* 1997;22A:1016–1024.

Ochiai N, Matsui T, Miyaji N, et al. Vascular anatomy of flexor tendons. I. Vincular systems and blood supply of the profundus tendon in the digital sheath. *J Hand Surg.* 1979;4:321–330.

Phillips CS, Falender R, Mass DP. The flexor synovial sheath of the little finger: a macroscopic study. *J Hand Surg.* 1995;20A:636–641.

Rayan GM. Palmar fascia complex anatomy and pathology in Dupuytren's disease. *Hand Clin.* 1999;15:73–86.

1.5   Intrinsic Musculature of the Hand

GENERAL

- Central axis of the hand is the long finger metacarpal/ray

Interosseous Muscles (Figs. 1.5-1 to 1.5-6)

- Originate from metacarpal diaphyses
- **"DAB"—Dorsal = ABDUCTION**
- **"PAD"—Palmar = ADDUCTION**
- Pass **dorsal** to the **deep transverse intermetacarpal ligament**
- **The deep transverse intermetacarpal ligament** connects the volar plates of the metacarpophalangeal joints of the index—long, ring, small—fingers and is continuous proximally with the fascia of the interosseous muscles of the hand. The distal margin of the ligament is approximately 2 cm proximal to the interdigital skin fold. The ligament is continuous with the ulnar collateral ligament of the small finger medially and the radial collateral ligament of the index finger laterally. The sagittal bands stabilizing the extensor mechanism insert into its dorsal surface and the A1 pulleys of the flexor retinacular system insert into its palmar surface. Structures palmar to the ligament include the flexor tendons, lumbrical muscles, and neurovascular bundles; however, the interossei pass dorsal to the ligament.
- Innervated by ulnar nerve
  - First IO may be innervated by median nerve through a Martin–Gruber (forearm) or Riche–Cannieu (hand) interconnection.

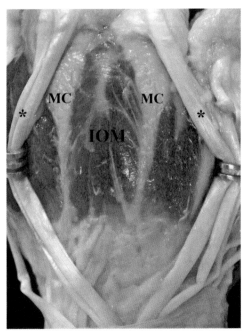

FIGURE 1.5-1 Dorsal view of the hand with retraction of the extrinsic digital extensor tendons *(*)* and exposure of the dorsal interosseous muscles *(IOM)*. The IOM take their origin from the periosteal margins of the metacarpals *(MC)*.

Dorsal Interossei

- Four dorsal interossei
- Bipennate; arise from both metacarpals of intermetacarpal space
- Each dorsal IO has two muscle bellies:

  Superficial

- Passes *under* sagittal hood to become **medial tendon**
- Insertion: **lateral tubercle of proximal phalanx**
- Action: **abductor of digit**

  Deep

- Passes *over* sagittal hood to become **lateral tendon**
- Insertion: **transverse fibers of extensor apparatus**
- Action: **flexor of MCP joint**

Volar Interossei

- Three volar interossei
- **Unipennate**; arises on metacarpal of same digit into which it inserts
- Insertion: **extensor apparatus on adductor side of digit**
- **No insertion into proximal phalanx**
- Action: flexor of MCP joint and adductor of index, ring, and small

LUMBRICAL MUSCLES (Figs. 1.5-2 and 1.5-3)

- Originate from **FDP tendon**
- Passes **volar** to the deep transverse intermetacarpal ligament
- Located on the radial side of each digit

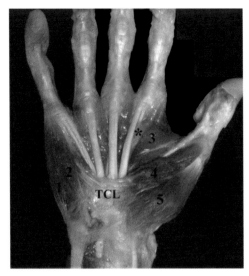

FIGURE 1.5-2 Palmar and superficial exposure of the intrinsic muscles of the hand. The transverse carpal ligament *(TCL)* serves as an origin for the flexor digiti minimi (FDM) *(2)*, the flexor pollicis brevis (FPB) *(4)*, and the abductor pollicis brevis (APB) *(5)*. The abductor digiti minimi (ADM) *(1)* originates at the distal pisiform and inserts at the ulnar base of the proximal phalanx and the extensor apparatus to the small finger. The radial and volar orientation of the lumbrical muscle *(*)* is identified relative to its origin along the flexor digitorum profundus tendon, its proximal attachment within or slightly distal to the distal segment of the carpal canal. The lumbrical muscle originates from and, therefore, may act to relax its own antagonist muscle (FDP). The adductor pollicis brevis muscle (ADD) *(3)* is seen deep to the thenar musculature, its broad origin along the volar and radial margin of the long finger metacarpal.

- Insertion: **radial lateral band (of extensor apparatus) via oblique fibers**
- Action: **extend PIP and DIP joints**
- Only muscle able to "relax" its antagonist (origin on FDP)
- Innervation:
  - First and second lumbricals (unipennate)
    - Median nerve
  - Second and third lumbricals (bipennate)
    - Ulnar nerve

THENAR MUSCLES

- Abductor pollicis brevis (APB)
  - Origin: transverse carpal ligament, FCR sheath, trapezium, scaphoid
  - Insertion: radial base P1, MCP joint capsule, radial sesamoid
  - Innervation: median (95%); ulnar (2.5%); both (2.5%)
  - Action: (i) abd + flexion of thumb metacarpal; (ii) ulnar angulation at MCP joint; (iii) thumb IP joint extension
- Flexor pollicis brevis (FPB)
  - Origin: transverse carpal ligament
  - Insertion: thumb MP joint capsule and radial sesamoid
  - Innervation: superficial head—median; deep head—ulnar
  - Action: (i) flexion of thumb metacarpal + P1; (ii) thumb pronation; (iii) thumb IP joint extension

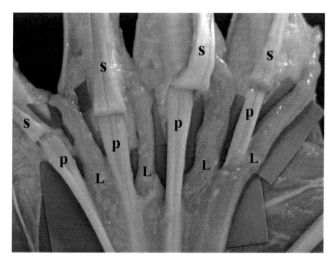

FIGURE 1.5-3 Palmar view of the flexor tendons and lumbrical origins. The flexor digitorum superficialis (FDS) tendons have been cut and reflected distally *(s)* to expose the FDP tendons *(p)* and the radial origin of each of the lumbrical muscles *(L)*.

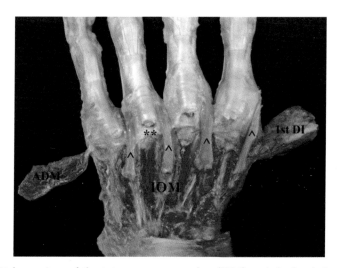

FIGURE 1.5-4 Palmar view of the interosseous muscles *(IOM)* and the lumbrical muscles *(^)* following removal of the extrinsic flexor tendons. The orientation of these intrinsic muscles relative to the deep transverse intermetacarpal ligament *(**)* is demonstrated; the lumbrical muscles remain palmar to the ligament with the digital neurovascular bundles while the interosseous muscles pass dorsal to the ligament.

- Opponens pollicis (OPP)
  - Origin: transverse carpal ligament, trapezium, thumb CMC capsule
  - Insertion: volar-radial distal thumb metacarpal
  - Innervation: median (83%); ulnar (10%); both (7%)
  - Action: (i) flexion and pronation of thumb metacarpal
- Adductor pollicis (ADD)
  - Origin: long finger metacarpal
  - Insertion: ulnar sesamoid of thumb, ulnar base of P1, dorsal apparatus
  - Innervation: ulnar nerve
  - Action: (i) adduction of thumb metacarpal; (ii) thumb IP joint extension

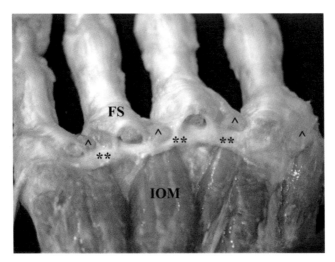

FIGURE 1.5-5 Proximal perspective of the lumbrical *(^)* and interosseous muscle *(IOM)* relationship relative to the deep transverse intermetacarpal ligament *(**)* is demonstrated. The lumbrical muscles remain palmar to the ligament with the digital neurovascular bundles and the interosseous muscles pass dorsal to the ligament. The flexor tendons have been cut and are contained distally within the flexor sheath *(FS)*.

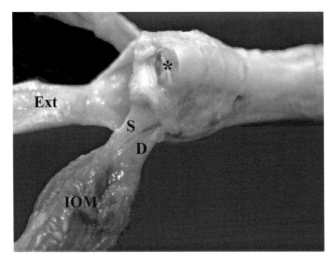

FIGURE 1.5-6 Single digit exposure of the dorsal interosseous tendon *(IOM)* insertion. The lumbrical muscle and deep transverse intermetacarpal ligament have been resected. The superficial head *(S)* passes under the sagittal hood to become the medial tendon and to insert into the lateral tubercle of the proximal phalanx. The deep head *(D)* of the dorsal interosseous muscle passes over the sagittal hood to become the lateral tendon and to insert into the transverse fibers of the extensor apparatus. Note that the volar interosseous does not insert into the proximal phalanx; its insertion is into the extensor apparatus only. The extensor tendon *(Ext)* and flexor tendon within the flexor sheath *(*)* are identified for reference.

HYPOTHENAR MUSCLES

- Palmaris brevis
- Abductor digiti minimi (ADM)
  - Origin: distal pisiform, FCU insertion
  - Insertion: ulnar base P1 (90%) and extensor apparatus (10%)

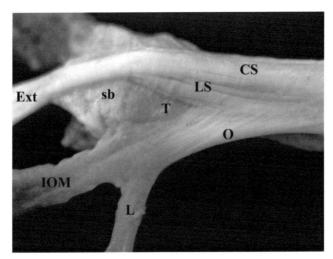

FIGURE 1.5-7 The dorsal digital extensor apparatus is derived from contributions of the extrinsic extensor tendons and the intrinsic musculature of the hand. The extrinsic extensor tendon *(Ext)* is identified at the level of the distal hand and splits into two lateral slips *(LS)* and the central tendon slip *(CS)*. At the dorsal MCP joint, the extensor tendon is stabilized by the vertically orientated fibers of the sagittal band *(sb)*, which originate from the radial and ulnar sides of the volar plate of the MCP joint and the volar base of the proximal phalanx. The MCP joint is extended via a sling-like mechanism of the sagittal band as there is no direct fiber insertion from the extrinsic extensor tendon at the proximal phalanx. The deep head of the interosseous muscle *(IOM)* courses superficial to the sagittal band *(sb)* at the level of the MCP joint and runs parallel and distal to the sagittal band over the proximal phalanx to form the transverse fibers *(T)* of the extensor apparatus. The lumbrical muscle *(L)* on the radial aspect of the digit forms the oblique fibers *(O)* of the extensor apparatus, which join with the lateral slip of the extrinsic extensor tendon to form the conjoined lateral band *(CLB)*.

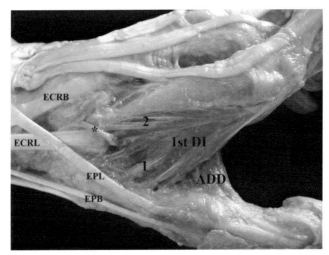

FIGURE 1.5-8 Oblique view of the first webspace demonstrating the relationships of the dorsal extrinsic and intrinsic musculature acting on the thumb and index finger. The first dorsal interosseous muscle *(1st DI)* originates from fibers attaching at both the index *(2)* and the thumb metacarpals *(1)*. The radial artery is identified *(*)* as it penetrates the interval between these two heads of the 1st DI. The adductor pollicis muscle *(ADD)* is located palmar to the 1st DI, and it inserts into the ulnar sesamoid, the ulnar base of the thumb proximal phalanx, and into the dorsal apparatus of the thumb. The extensor carpi radialis longus *(ECRL)* and brevis *(ECRB)* insert into the dorsal base of the index and long fingers, respectively. The extensor pollicis longus *(EPL)* tendon is ulnar to the inserting extensor pollicis brevis *(EPB)* tendon and functions to extend the thumb interphalangeal joint, but also to adduct the thumb based on its orientation.

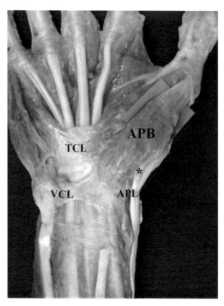

FIGURE 1.5-9 Palmar view of the abductor pollicis brevis muscle *(APB)* and its relationships. The APB originates from the transverse carpal ligament *(TCL)* and inserts into the radial base of the thumb proximal phalanx, the thumb MP joint capsule, and the radial sesamoid of the thumb. The extrinsic abductor pollicis longus tendon *(APL)* is seen inserting, in part, into the APB muscle *(*)*. The flexor pollicis brevis and adductor pollicis muscles are dorsal to the APB. The volar carpal ligament (VCL) extends from the TCL radially to cover the ulnar neurovascular bundle, as the roof of the distal ulnar tunnel, or Guyon's canal.

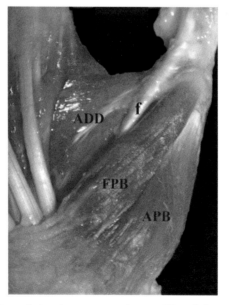

FIGURE 1.5-10 Palmar view of the thenar musculature. The abductor pollicis brevis *(APB)* and the flexor pollicis brevis *(FPB)* muscles originate from the transverse carpal ligament; the FPB origin is more distal than that of the APB. The flexor pollicis longus tendon *(f)* emerges from the interval between the deeper adductor pollicis *(ADD)* muscle and the FPB/APB.

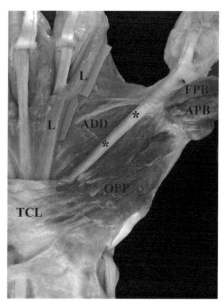

FIGURE 1.5-11 Palmar view of the deep thenar musculature relationships after distal reflection of the FPB and APB muscles. The opponens pollicis *(OPP)* originates from the transverse carpal ligament *(TCL)*, the trapezium, and the thumb CMC joint capsule, and it inserts into the volar-radial distal thumb metacarpal. The OPP muscle acts to flex and pronate the thumb metacarpal. The flexor pollicis longus tendon *(*)* is seen to emerge from the carpal canal to run radially on the palmar surface of the adductor pollicis muscle *(ADD)*, deep to the OPP muscle. The lumbrical muscle to the index finger *(L)* is identified at its origin along the radial and volar margins of the flexor digitorum profundus tendon to the index finger.

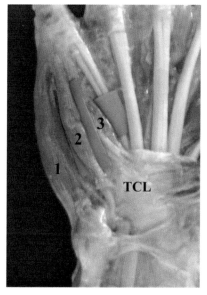

FIGURE 1.5-12 Palmar view of the hypothenar eminence, subdivided into its components: abductor digiti minimi (ADM) *(1)*, flexor digiti minimi (FDM) *(2)*, and opponens digiti minimi (ODM) *(3)*. The ADM origin is the distal pisiform and FCU insertion, whereas both the FDM and the ODM originate from the transverse carpal ligament *(TCL)* and the hook of the hamate.

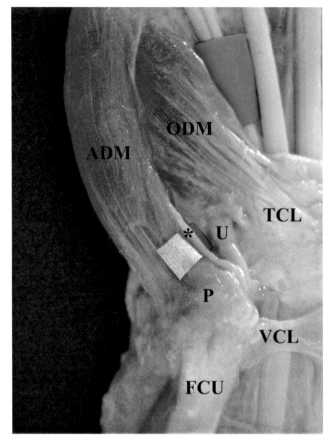

FIGURE 1.5-13 Close-up palmar view of the abductor digiti minimi *(ADM)* and the opponens digiti minimi *(ODM)* after removal of the flexor digiti minimi muscle. The course of the ulnar nerve *(U)* is identified from its position deep and radial to the flexor carpi ulnaris tendon *(FCU)* to emerge from the distal ulnar tunnel at the distal edge of the pisiform *(P)*. The ulnar nerve is deep to the volar carpal ligament *(VCL)* and superficial to the transverse carpal ligament *(TCL)*. The ulnar nerve sends a motor branch to the ADM *(*)* before piercing the ODM to traverse the palm in a radial direction to innervate the deep intrinsic muscles of the hand.

- Innervation: ulnar nerve
- Action: (i) strong abductor of small finger; (ii) mild MCP joint flexion of small; (iii) small finger IP joint extension
- Flexor digiti minimi (FDM)
  - Origin: transverse carpal ligament, hook of hamate
  - Insertion: small finger P1 palmar base
  - Innervation: ulnar nerve
  - Action: (i) small finger flexion at MP joint absent in 15% to 20% of hands
- Opponens digiti minimi (ODM)
  - Origin: transverse carpal ligament, hook of hamate
  - Insertion: distal three-fourth ulnar aspect of small metacarpal
  - Innervation: ulnar nerve
  - Action: (i) small metacarpal supination; (ii) deepens palm to complement thumb opposition

■ *Clinical Correlate:* Testing of the first dorsal interosseous muscle is done with the index MCP joint in 30° to 40° flexion to negate potential influence of the extrinsic extensors.

RECOMMENDED READING

Al-Qattan MM, Robertson GA. An anatomical study of the deep transverse metacarpal ligament. *J Anat*. 1993;182:443–446.

Eladoumikdachi F, Valkov PL, Thomas J, et al. Anatomy of the intrinsic hand muscles revisited, part I: interossei. *Plast Reconstr Surg*. 2002;110:1211–1224.

Eladoumikdachi F, Valkov PL, Thomas J, et al. Anatomy of the intrinsic hand muscles revisited, part II: lumbricals. *Plast Reconstr Surg*. 2002;110:1225–1231.

Eyler DL, Markee JE. The anatomy and function of the intrinsic musculature of the fingers. *J Bone Joint Surg*. 1954;36A:1–9.

Kanaya K, Wada T, Isogai S, et al. Variation in insertion of the abductor digiti minimi: an anatomic study. *J Hand Surg*. 2002;27A:325–328.

Smith RJ. Intrinsic muscles of the fingers: function, dysfunction, and surgical reconstruction. In: *AAOS Instructional Course Lecture*, vol. 24. St. Louis, MO: C. V. Mosby; 1975: 200–220.

von Schroeder HP, Botte MJ. The dorsal aponeurosis, intrinsic, hypothenar, and thenar musculature of the hand. *Clin Orthop Relat Res*. 2001;383:97–107.

1.6   Cross-Sectional Anatomy of the Hand

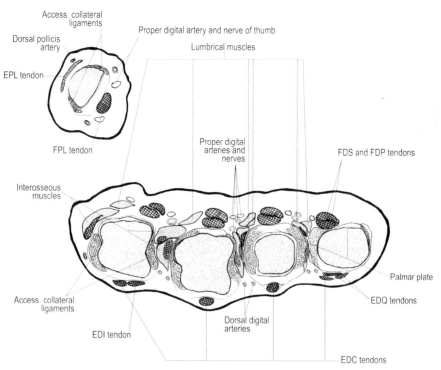

FIGURE 1.6-1 Illustration of cross-sectional anatomy at the level of the finger metacarpophalangeal (MCP) joints. Note the relationship of the intrinsic muscles of the hand to the palmar plate of the MCP joints. The lumbrical muscles and digital neurovascular bundles pass palmar to the deep transverse intermetacarpal ligament (not shown), whereas the interossei are located dorsal to the ligament. Unlike the fingers that rely on the digital arteries for both volar and dorsal vascular perfusion, the thumb has both a dorsal and a volar arterial supply.

2 Wrist

2.1 Osteology and Joints of the Wrist

DISTAL RADIUS AND ULNA (Figs. 2.1-1 to 2.1-3)

- The distal radius articular surface has two concave facets, the **scaphoid and lunate facets**, separated by the **scapholunate or anterior–posterior ridge**.
- The dorsal distal radius is **dihedral** in shape. Relative to the dorsal cortex of the distal radius, Lister's tubercle projects dorsally (2 to 6 mm) and the EPL groove may be 1 to 5 mm in depth.
- The **sigmoid notch**, along the ulnar border of the distal radius, is a shallow concavity for the articulating ulnar head.
- Actual contact area of the articular surfaces is between 10% and 60%.
- The distal ulna is covered with hyaline cartilage on its dorsal, lateral, palmar, and distal surfaces.
- The ulnar styloid projects distally; at its base, the **fovea** is a recessed, nonarticulating site that is the insertion for the TFCC.

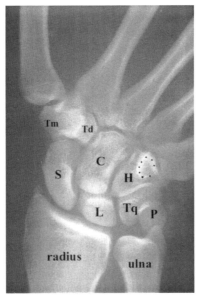

FIGURE 2.1-1 Posteroanterior radiograph of the right wrist in ulnar deviation. Note the elongated appearance of the scaphoid *(S)* (extended). Lunate *(L)*, triquetrum *(Tq)*, pisiform *(P)*, hamate *(H)*, capitate *(C)*, trapezoid *(Td)*, and trapezium *(Tm)*. Note the outlined cortical profile of the hook of the hamate *(. . .)* that projects in the posteroanterior plane.

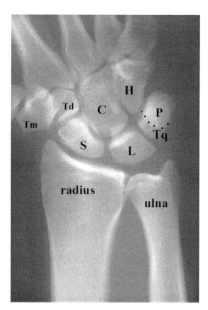

FIGURE 2.1-2 Posteroanterior radiograph of the right wrist in radial deviation. Note the fore-shortened appearance of the scaphoid *(S)* (flexed). Lunate *(L)*, triquetrum *(Tq)*, pisiform *(P)*, hamate *(H)*, capitate *(C)*, trapezoid *(Td)*, and trapezium *(Tm)*. Note the outlined cortical profile of the pisiform *(. . .)* that overlaps with the triquetrum.

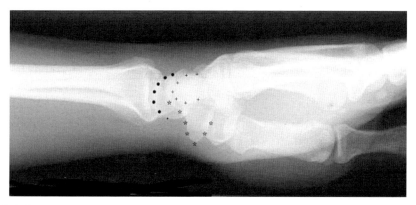

FIGURE 2.1-3 Lateral radiographic view of the wrist. The profiles of the proximal lunate *(. . .)*, proximal–palmar scaphoid *(***)*, and proximal capitate *(+ + +)* are outlined.

CARPUS

- Eight ossicles separated, traditionally, into **proximal** (scaphoid, lunate, triquetrum, pisiform) and **distal** (trapezium, trapezoid, capitate, hamate) **carpal rows**.

Scaphoid

- Primary vascular supply from branch of radial artery at dorsal ridge supplies approximately 70% of the scaphoid.
- A group of smaller vessels enters the palmar tubercle and supplies the distal 30%.
- The transverse carpal ligament attaches to the palmar tubercle.
- The distal-dorsal surface serves as an attachment site for the dorsal intercarpal ligament (DIC).

Lunate

- Dorsal + palmar vascular supply in 80%; palmar only in 20%
- Broader palmarly than dorsally
- Type I lunate does not have a medial facet for articulation with the hamate; a Type II lunate has a medial hamate facet.

Triquetrum

- Site of attachment for the meniscal homolog of the TFCC
- Palmar surface has an oval facet for articulation with the pisiform.
- Dorsal surface: origin of the DIC and insertion of DRC

Hamate

- Body and hook (hamulus) of hamate
- The hook of the hamate serves as an attachment for the transverse carpal ligament and for the origins of the flexor digiti minimi and opponens digiti minimi
- Distal surface articulates with the bases of the ring and small finger metacarpals via two articular facets; facets are separated by an scapholunate ridge.

Capitate

- Head (proximal) often relies on a retrograde vascular supply.
- Two ridges separate the distal articular surface into three facets for articulation with the index, long, ring metacarpals.

Trapezoid

- Two distal facets that articulate with the index metacarpal and the trapezium

Trapezium

- Saddle-shaped articulation with the thumb metacarpal base
- Additional articulations with the trapezoid and the index metacarpal base
- Palmar FCR groove, bordered laterally by a palmar tuberosity and the distal radial attachment of the transverse carpal ligament

Pisiform

- Sesamoid bone within FCU tendon
- One origin of the abductor digiti minimi

OSSEOUS DEVELOPMENT (Fig. 2.1-4)

Radiographic appearance of carpal ossification centers:
- Capitate (3 to 6 months)
- Hamate (4 to 8 months)
- Triquetrum (2 to 3 years)
- Lunate (4 years)
- Scaphoid (4 to 5 years)
- Trapezium (5 years)
- Trapezoid (6 years)
- Pisiform (6 to 8 years)

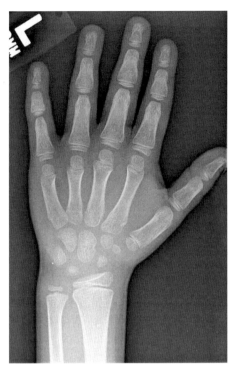

FIGURE 2.1-4 Posteroanterior radiograph of the left wrist of an 8-year-old male. Note the ossification centers of each of the carpus and the open physes of the distal radius and ulna. The physis of the thumb metacarpal is at its base, unlike those of the finger metacarpals that are distal.

DEVELOPMENTAL ANOMALIES OF THE CARPUS AND PHALANGES

- **Kirner deformity**: a palmar and radial curvature of the small finger distal phalanx
- **Clinodactyly**: typically involves a short middle phalanx of the small finger and mild radial deviation of the distal phalanx, possibly associated with hypoplasia of the radial aspect of the middle phalanx
- **Delta phalanx**: asymmetric development of a secondary ossification center within the phalanx; results in the formation of a triangular-shaped bone, linking the proximal and distal epiphyses, with a continuous physis or epiphysis along its shorter side. Can contribute to clinodactyly.
- Accessory ossicles: over 25 have been described
- Most common carpal coalition: (1) **lunotriquetral** and (2) capitohamate
- **Madelung deformity**: congenital dyschondrosteosis primarily involving the ulnar portion of the distal radial physis and adjacent bony epiphysis. Dysplasia of the ulnar column results in a palmar and ulnar inclination of the ulnar articular surface with resultant shortening and bowing of the radius.

RECOMMENDED READING

af Ekenstam F, Hagert CG. Anatomical studies on the geometry and stability of the distal radioulnar joint. *Scand J Plast Reconstr Surg.* 1985;19:17.

Berger RA. The anatomy of the scaphoid. *Hand Clin.* 2001;17:525–532.

Bugbee WB, Botte MJ. Surface anatomy of the hand. The relationships between palmar skin creases and osseous anatomy. *Clin Orthop Relat Res.* 1993;296:122–126.

Canovas F, Roussanne Y, Captier G, et al. Study of carpal bone morphology and position in three dimensions by image analysis from computed tomography scans of the wrist. *Surg Radiol Anat.* 2004;26:186–190. [Epub 2004, May 7].

Clement H, Pichler W, Nelson D, et al. Morphometric analysis of Lister's tubercle and its consequences on volar plate fixation of distal radius fractures. *J Hand Surg.* 2008;33A: 1716–1719.

Freedman DM, Botte MJ, Gelberman RH. Vascularity of the carpus. *Clin Orthop Relat Res.* 2001; 383:47–59.

Gelberman RH, Menon J. The vascularity of the scaphoid bone. *J Hand Surg.* 1980;5A: 508–513.

Greulich WW, Pyle SI. *Radiographic Atlas of Skeletal Development of the Hand and Wrist.* 2nd ed. Stanford, CA: Stanford University Press; 1959.

Handley RC, Pooley J. The venous anatomy of the scaphoid. *J Anat.* 1991;178:115–118.

Jayasekera N, Akhtar N, Compson JP. Physical examination of the carpal bones by orthopaedic and accident and emergency surgeons. *J Hand Surg.* 2005;30B:204–206.

Mayfield JK, Johnson RP, Kilcoyne RK. Carpal dislocations: pathomechanics and progressive perilunar instability. *J Hand Surg.* 1980;5:226–241.

Panagis JS, Gelberman RH, Taleisnik J, et al. The arterial anatomy of the human carpus. Part II: the intraosseous vascularity. *J Hand Surg.* 1983;8A:375–382.

Placzek JD, Sobol GV, Arnoczky SP, et al. The effect of an extended flexor carpi radialis approach on blood flow to the distal radius: a cadaveric study. *Orthopaedics.* 2005;28:1364–1367.

Spielmann PM, Oliver CW. The carpal bones: a basic test of medical students' and junior doctors' knowledge of anatomy. *Surgeon.* 2005;3:257–259.

Vander Grend R, Dell PC, Glowczewskie F, et al. Intraosseous blood supply of the capitate and its correlation with aseptic necrosis. *J Hand Surg.* 1984;9A:677–683.

2.2   Ligamentous Anatomy of the Wrist

EXTRINSIC WRIST LIGAMENTS—VOLAR

Radiocarpal

- **Radial collateral (RCL)**
  Variable presence
  Origin: radius (0 mm from radial styloid tip)
  Insertion: scaphoid waist and distal palmar trapezium
- **Radioscaphocapitate (RSC)**
  Origin: radius (4 mm from radial styloid tip)
  Insertion: scaphoid waist + midpalmar capitate
- **Long radiolunate (LRL)**
  Origin: radius (10 mm from radial styloid tip)
  Insertion: lunate ± triquetrum
- **Radioscapholunate (RSL)** also known as the ***ligament of Testut–Kuenz***
  Mesocapsule with termination of AIN + AIA
  Lies dorsal to the LRL ligament
  Origin: small tubercle on volar lip of distal radius
  Insertion: primarily into lunate; secondarily into scaphoid
- **Short radiolunate (short RL)**
  Origin: volar–ulnar margin of radius
  Insertion: lunate (ulnar margin of palmar horn)

Ulnocarpal (Figs. 2.2-1 and 2.2-2)

- **Ulnotriquetral (UT)**
  Origin: volar radioulnar ligament
  Insertion: triquetrum
- **Ulnolunate (UL)**
  Origin: volar radioulnar ligament
  Insertion: lunate

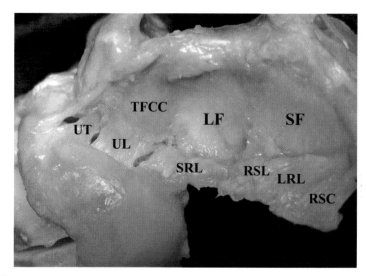

FIGURE 2.2-1 End-on view of the right distal radius articular surface and the ulnocarpal joint with the carpus reflected palmarly and ulnarly. The scaphoid facet *(SF)* and lunate facet *(LF)* of the distal radius are separated by the scapholunate ridge. The volar extrinsic ligaments originate from the distal radius and include the radioscaphocapitate *(RSC)*, long radiolunate *(LRL)*, radioscapholunate *(RSL)*, and short radiolunate *(SRL)* ligaments. Components of the TFCC include: (i) central meniscal homolog *(TFCC)*; (ii) dorsal and volar radioulnar ligaments (not shown); (iii) ulnolunate ligament *(UL)*; (iv) ulnotriquetral ligament *(UT)*; (v) floor of the ECU sheath (not shown).

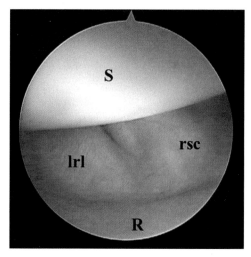

FIGURE 2.2-2 Arthroscopic visualization of the radioscaphoid joint (*R*, radius; *S*, scaphoid) of the right wrist. The oblique orientations of the radioscaphocapitate ligament *(rsc)* and the long radiolunate ligament *(lrl)* are appreciated through the 3–4 portal (see Section 2.4).

- **Ulnocapitate (UC)**
    Origin: volar margin ulnar head
    Insertion: capitate
  ➢ Note that the UC ligament is the only ulnocarpal ligament to attach to the ulnar head; the UT and UL ligaments attach at the volar radioulnar ligament, a component of the TFCC.

■ *Clinical Correlate:* The space of Poirier is described at the volar aspect of the capitolunate joint between the RSC and LRL ligaments. This interligamentous space becomes more defined with increasing extension of the wrist and is the site of lunate dislocation in progressive perilunate instability.

EXTRINSIC WRIST LIGAMENTS—DORSAL (Fig. 2.2-3)

- **Dorsal radiocarpal (DRC)**
    Origin: dorsal lip of distal radius; origin roughly of equal size from each side of Lister's tubercle
    Insertion: radial fibers into lunate + lunotriquetral interosseous ligament; terminal insertion into dorsal tubercle of triquetrum
- **Dorsal intercarpal (DIC)**
    Origin: dorsal tubercle of triquetrum
    Insertion: lunate + dorsal groove of scaphoid ± capitate ± trapezium ± trapezoid

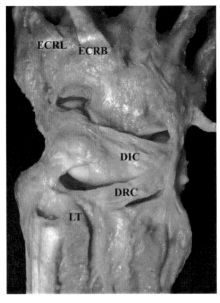

FIGURE 2.2-3 Dorsal view of the right wrist with the extensor carpi radialis longus and brevis (**ECRL** and **ECRB**) reflected distally. The dorsal extrinsic wrist ligaments are identified. The dorsal radiocarpal ligament *(DRC)* originates at the dorsal lip of the distal radius, adjacent to the dorsal radial tubercle or Lister's tubercle *(LT)*. It traverses the radiocarpal joint obliquely to insert into the lunate and the dorsal tubercle of the triquetrum. The dorsal intercarpal ligament *(DIC)* arises from the dorsal tubercle of the triquetrum and inserts into the lunate, the distal dorsal scaphoid, and occasionally the trapezoid and capitate.

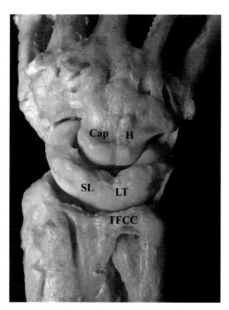

FIGURE 2.2-4 Dorsal view of the right wrist after resection of the extrinsic ligaments. The dorsal aspect of the *TFCC* (dorsal radioulnar ligament) is visualized. The scapholunate interosseous ligament *(SL)* and lunotriquetral interosseous ligament *(LT)* stabilize the proximal *carpal* row. The capitate *(Cap)* and hamate *(H)* are identified in the distal carpal row.

INTRINSIC WRIST LIGAMENTS (Fig. 2.2-4)

- **Scapholunate interosseous ligament (SL)**
  - C-shaped, in sagittal plane
  - Dorsal 1/3 thickest, most important stabilizer
- **Lunotriquetral interosseous ligament (LT)**
  - Volar: thickest

■ *Clinical Correlate:* Disruption of the scapholunate interosseous ligament and associated radiocarpal ligaments leads to abnormal flexion of the scaphoid and extension of the lunate. A scapholunate advanced collapse (SLAC) wrist will develop with time; progressive arthrosis of the wrist occurs beginning at the radiocarpal joint and advancing to include the midcarpal joints.

■ *Clinical Correlate:* Disruption of the lunotriquetral interosseous ligament may result in the development of excessive lunate flexion (a VISI deformity) and a concomitant midcarpal extension deformity leading to decreased range of motion, weakness, and pain.

TRIANGULAR FIBROCARTILAGENOUS COMPLEX (TFCC) (Fig. 2.2-5)

- Formed by:
  - **Triangular fibrocartilage proper—articular disc**
  - **Ulnocarpal meniscus homolog**
  - **Dorsal and volar radioulnar ligaments**
  - **Floor of ECU tendon sheath**
  - **Volar ulnocarpal ligaments**

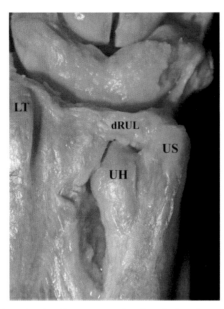

FIGURE 2.2-5 The dorsal distal radioulnar joint. The distal ulna (*UH*, ulnar head; *US*, ulnar styloid) articulates with the distal radius at the distal radioulnar joint where the distal radial articular surface (sigmoid notch) has a greater radius of curvature than that of the ulnar head. The DRUJ is constrained by the dorsal *(dRUL)* and volar (not seen) distal radioulnar ligaments. The distal radioulnar ligaments are components of the TFCC. Lister's tubercle *(LT)* is identified for reference.

- Arises from radial border of distal radius and inserts at the fovea at the base of the ulnar styloid
- Biconcave in shape; it articulates with the head of the ulna proximally and primarily the triquetrum distally.
- The **prestyloid synovial recess** at the tip of the ulnar styloid is found between the meniscus and the triangular fibrocartilage.
- The **dorsal and volar radioulnar ligaments** are primary stabilizers of the DRUJ.
- The proximal components, or limbi, of the dorsal and volar radioulnar ligaments conjoin to insert into the fovea and are referred to as the **ligamentum subcruentum**.
- The distal components, or limbi, of the dorsal and volar radioulnar ligaments insert directly into the base of the ulnar styloid, independent of the insertion of the proximal limbi.
- Dorsally, the TFCC is stabilized to the ulnar carpus through the ECU sheath.
- The ulnocarpal meniscus homolog is a layer of thickened fibrous connective tissue, confluent with the fibers arising from the ulnar styloid (ulnar collateral ligament) and fibers that insert broadly into the triquetrum, hamate, and small finger metacarpal base.
- The vascular supply is limited to the **peripheral 10% to 40%** of the volar, ulnar, and dorsal TFCC only.

■ *Clinical Correlate:* Typically, TFCC repairs are performed for peripheral ulnar or dorsal–ulnar tears with a high expectation for healing. Radial-sided tears may be repaired. Central TFCC tears are not repaired, but often are debrided to create a "stable" tear.

■ *Clinical Correlate:* The extrinsic and intrinsic ligaments of the wrist are often more clearly identified and evaluated from within the joint, such as with wrist arthroscopy.

CARPAL KINEMATICS

- Proximal carpal row has no muscular or tendinous attachments and is an intercalary segment.
- **Ulnar deviation**: (approximately 30°) proximal row **extends** relative to the forearm/distal row (scaphoid extension, lunate extension, and "hamate-low" position).
- **Radial deviation**: (approximately 20°) proximal row **flexes** relative to the forearm/distal row (scaphoid flexion, lunate flexion, and "hamate-high" position).
- **Force distribution**: approximately 80% of forces are transmitted through the distal radius (60% scaphoid facet/40% lunate facet)/20% distal ulna with axial loading through the neutral wrist.
- **Wrist flexion**: (approximately 80°) 60% midcarpal/40% radiocarpal motion
- **Wrist extension**: (approximately 70°) 33% midcarpal 66% radiocarpal motion

RECOMMENDED READING

Bednar MS, Arnoczky SP, Weiland AJ. The microvasculature of the triangular fibrocartilage complex: its clinical significance. *J Hand Surg*. 1991;16A:1101–1105.

Berger RA. The gross and histologic anatomy of the scapholunate interosseous ligament. *J Hand Surg*. 1996;20:170–178.

Berger RA, Blair WF, Crowninshield RD, et al. The scapholunate ligament. *J Hand Surg*. 1982;7:87–91.

Berger RA, Kauer JMG, Landsmeer JMF. Radioscapholunate ligament: a gross anatomic and histologic study of fetal and adult wrists. *J Hand Surg*. 1991;16A:350–355.

Berger RA, Landsmeer JM. The palmar radiocarpal ligaments: a study of adult and fetal human wrist joints. *J Hand Surg*. 1990;15A:847–854.

Elsaidi GA, Ruch DS, Kuzma GR, et al. Dorsal wrist ligament insertions stabilize the scapholunate interval: cadaver study. *Clin Orthop Relat Res*. 2004;425:152–157.

Garcia-Elias M, Domenech-Mateu JM. The articular disc of the wrist: limits and relations. *Acta Anat*. 1987;128:51.

Kauer JMG, de Lange A. The carpal joint: anatomy and function. *Hand Clin*. 1987;3:23–29.

Mayfield JK, Johnson RP, Kilcoyne RK. The ligaments of the human wrist and their functional significance. *Anat Rec*. 1976;186:417–428.

Mayfield JK, Johnson RP, Kilcoyne RK. Carpal dislocations: pathomechanics and progressive perilunar instability. *J Hand Surg*. 1980;5:226–241.

Nakamura T, Takayama S, Horiuchi Y, et al. Origins and insertions of the triangular fibrocartilage complex: a histological study. *J Hand Surg*. 2001;26B:446–454.

Nishikawa S, Toh S. Anatomical study of the carpal attachment of the triangular fibrocartilage complex. *J Bone Joint Surg*. 2002;84(B):1062–1065.

Palmer AK, Werner FW. The triangular fibrocartilage complex of the wrist—anatomy and function. *J Hand Surg*. 1981;6:153–162.

Sennwald GR, Zdravkovic V, Oberlin C. The anatomy of the palmar scaphotriquetral ligament. *J Bone Joint Surg*. 1994;76B:147–149.

Siegel DB, Gelberman RH. Radial styloidectomy: an anatomical study with special reference to radiocarpal intracapsular ligamentous morphology. *J Hand Surg*. 1991;16A: 40–44.

Sokolow C, Saffar P. Anatomy and histology of the scapholunate ligament. *Hand Clin*. 2001;17: 77–81.

Taleisnik J. The ligaments of the wrist. *J Hand Surg*. 1976;1:110–118.

Viegas SF. The dorsal ligaments of the wrist. *Hand Clin*. 2001;17:65–75.

Viegas SF, Yamaguchi S, Boyd NL, et al. The dorsal ligaments of the wrist: anatomy, mechanical properties, and function. *J Hand Surg*. 1999;24:456–468.

| **2.3** | **Cross-Sectional Anatomy of the Wrist** |

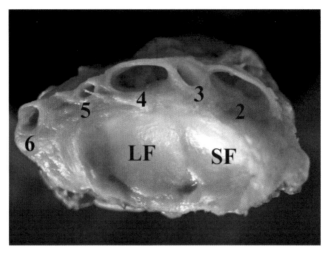

FIGURE 2.3-1 Axial view of the right distal radius articular surface and TFCC after soft tissue removal. The extensor retinaculum and the vertical septa have been preserved to appreciate the second to sixth extensor compartments at the level of the wrist. Note that the fifth extensor compartment (extensor digitorum minimi/quinti) overlies the distal radioulnar joint (*SF*, scaphoid fossa; *LF*, lunate fossa; *2*, second extensor compartment containing ECRL and ECRB; *3*, third extensor compartment with EPL; *4*, fourth extensor compartment with EDC and EIP; *5*, fifth extensor compartment with EDM/EDQ; *6*, sixth extensor compartment with ECU).

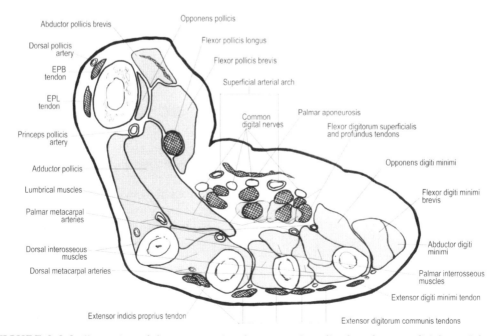

FIGURE 2.3-2 Illustration of the cross-sectional anatomy just distal to the superficial arterial arch at the wrist.

2.4 Arthroscopic Anatomy of the Wrist

DORSAL WRIST PORTALS

- Dorsal wrist portals are defined by their relationship to the extensor compartments.
- Structures at risk during portal access include:
    - Extensor tendons
    - Sensory branch of the radial nerve (SBRN)
    - Dorsal sensory branch of the ulnar nerve (DSBUN)
    - Radial artery (deep branch)

1–2 Portal

- Located between the first (APL + EPB) and second (ECR) extensor compartments
- Deep branch of the radial artery (1 to 5 mm from portal) and SBRN branches (1 to 6 mm) at greatest risk

3–4 Portal

- Approximately 8 to 10 mm distal to Lister's tubercle, between the third (EPL) and fourth (EDC–EIP) compartments
- The portal is directed slightly volar and proximal in order to account for the volar tilt of the normal distal radius and contour of the carpus.
- One branch of the SBRN may be at risk (5 to 22 mm).

4–5 Portal

- Between the fourth (EDC–EIP) and fifth (EDQ) tendon compartments
- Sensory nerves are generally at minimal risk for injury.

6R Portal

- Located on the radial side of the sixth extensor compartment, between the ECU and the EDQ tendons
- The DSBUN is in close proximity, particularly the transverse branch of the DSBUN (0 to 6 mm from portal).

6U Portal

- Located on the ulnar side of the sixth extensor compartment, ulnar to the ECU tendon
- The DSBUN is the structure at risk (1 to 4 mm from portal).

Distal Radioulnar Joint Portal (Dorsal)

- With the wrist in neutral rotation or in pronation, the portal is located between the fourth (EDC–EIP) and fifth (EDQ) or between the fifth (EDQ) and sixth (ECU) compartments.

Radial Midcarpal Portal

- Found between the ECRB (second extensor compartment) and the EDC (fourth extensor compartment), approximately 1 cm distal to the 3–4 portal
- The SBRN branches are at risk (2 to 12 mm from portal).

Ulnar Midcarpal Portal

- Located between the tendons of the fourth and fifth (EDQ) extensor compartments
- Branches of both SBRN and DSBUN may be at risk.

VOLAR WRIST PORTALS (Figs. 2.4-1 to 2.4-6)

Volar Radial Portal

- Mini-open incision in the FCR–radial artery interval; portal is created between long radiolunate and radioscapholunate ligaments.
- Good visualization of palmar portion of scapholunate interosseous ligament and origin of the dorsal radiocarpal ligament
- Structures at risk: radial artery, palmar cutaneous branch of the median nerve, and median nerve

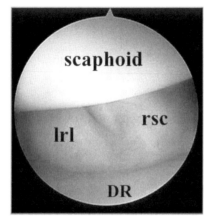

FIGURE 2.4-1 Wrist arthroscopy: view of the volar and radial aspects of the radiocarpal joint demonstrating the distal radius *(DR)*, the radioscaphocapitate ligament *(rsc)*, and the long radiolunate ligament *(lrl)*.

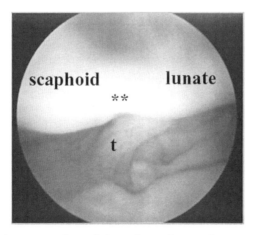

FIGURE 2.4-2 Wrist arthroscopy: view of the volar and central aspects of the radiocarpal joint. The scapholunate ligament *(**)* is distinguished from the scaphoid and lunate as a slight depression between the two bones (t, ligament of Testut).

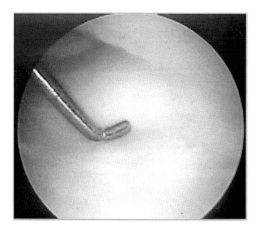

FIGURE 2.4-3 Wrist arthroscopy: view of the triangular fibrocartilagenous complex (TFCC) as identified by the probe.

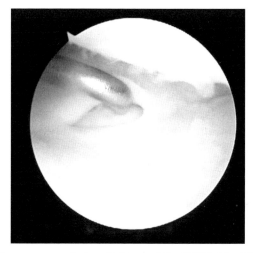

FIGURE 2.4-4 Wrist arthroscopy: central–radial tear of the TFCC, identified by the probe.

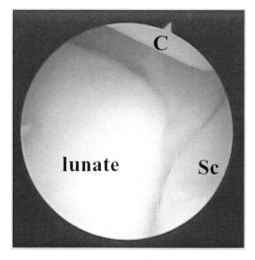

FIGURE 2.4-5 Wrist arthroscopy: midcarpal view of the scaphoid *(Sc)*, lunate, and capitate *(C)*.

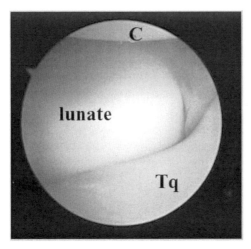

FIGURE 2.4-6 Wrist arthroscopy: midcarpal view of the lunate, triquetrum *(Tq)*, and capitate *(C)*.

Volar Ulnar Portal

- Mini-open incision along ulnar border of finger flexors, radial to ulnar neurovascular bundle
- Structures at risk: ulnar nerve, ulnar artery, flexor tendons, and median nerve

Volar Distal Radioulnar Joint Portal

- Useful for assessment of the foveal attachment of the TFCC

RECOMMENDED READING

Abrams RA, Petersen M, Botte MJ. Arthroscopic portals of the wrist: an anatomic study. *J Hand Surg.* 1994;19A:940–944.

Berger RA. Arthroscopic anatomy of the wrist and distal radioulnar joint. *Hand Clin.* 1999;15: 393–413.

Slutsky DJ. Wrist arthroscopy through a volar radial portal. *Arthroscopy.* 2002;18:624–630.

Slutsky DJ. The use of a volar ulnar portal in wrist arthroscopy. *Arthroscopy.* 2004;20: 158–163.

3 Forearm

3.1 Forearm Osteology (Figs. 3.1-1 and 3.1-2)

- The radius and ulna are stabilized by their articulations at the elbow and wrist and by the interosseous ligament complex (**IOLC**)/interosseous membrane (IOM).
- The IOLC serves several functions:
  - A stabilizing ligamentous interconnection between radius and ulna (longitudinal and transverse forces)
  - Facilitates load transfer between radius and ulna
  - Supports forearm pronation and supination
  - Musculotendinous origin (see Sections 3.2 and 3.3)
- The IOM originates on the radius and inserts on the ulna.
- The volar IOLC is comprised of three fiber groups (proximal to distal):
  - **Proximal band**
    - Also termed the *oblique ligament*
    - Originates in same region as IOL origin and courses proximally to insert approximately 9.5 cm distal to distal tip of olecranon
    - Oriented 28° to ulnar axis
    - 4 mm in width

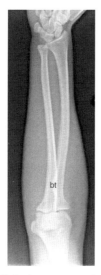

FIGURE 3.1-1 Anteroposterior radiograph of the forearm. The biceps tuberosity (bt) is identified.

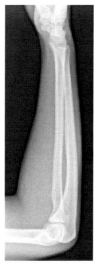

FIGURE 3.1-2 Lateral radiograph of the forearm.

- **IOL proper (central ligament)**
  - Width: 3.5 cm (measured along central forearm axis) or 2.6 cm (measured perpendicular to fiber orientation)
  - Thickness: approximately 1 mm
  - Originates approximately 7.7 cm distal to radial head and inserts into ulna approximately 13.7 cm distal to olecranon tip
  - Inserts into ulna at an approximately 21° orientation to longitudinal axis of forearm
- **Accessory bands**
  - Varies in number from 1 to 5
  - Distal to IOL proper, with similar fiber orientation

■ *Clinical Correlate:* In the absence of the radial head, the central ligament/band of the interosseous membrane is the primary stabilizer preventing proximal migration of the radius.

■ *Clinical Correlate:* In ulnar neutral variance, axial load through the wrist is distributed 80% through radiocarpal joint and 20% to ulna. The IOM serves to redistribute the axial forces such that, at the elbow, forces are measured 60% at the radiocapitellar joint and 40% at the ulnohumeral joint.

■ *Clinical Correlate:* An Essex–Lopresti injury involves a proximal radius fracture and concomitant soft tissue disruptions of the IOM and TFCC. Failure to recognize this injury may lead to longitudinal forearm dissociation.

RECOMMENDED READING

Green J, Zelouf DS. Forearm instability. *J Hand Surg.* 2009;34A:953–961.

Hotchkiss RN, An KA, Sowa DT, et al. An anatomic and mechanical study of the interosseous membrane of the forearm: pathomechanics of proximal migration of the radius. *J Hand Surg.* 1989;14A:256–261.

Marcotte AL, Osterman AL. Longitudinal radioulnar dissociation: identification and treatment of acute and chronic injuries. *Hand Clin.* 2007;23:195–208.

Skahan JR 3rd, Palmer AK, Werner FW, et al. The interosseous membrane of the forearm: anatomy and function. *J Hand Surg.* 1997;22A:981–985.

3.2   Dorsal Forearm

- Musculature may be considered in three groups:

Muscle	Origin	Insertion	Innervation
Mobile wad of three			
BR	Upper supracondylar ridge	Radial styloid	Radial nerve
ECRL	Lower supracondylar ridge	Radial base index metacarpal	Radial nerve
ECRB	Lateral epicondyle, elbow capsule, annular ligament	Radial base long metacarpal	SBRN (25%) + PIN (45%), radial nerve (30%)

(continued)

Muscle	Origin	Insertion	Innervation
Superficial extensor muscles			
Anconeus	Postlateral epicondyle	Lateral–dorsal ulna	Radial nerve
ECU	Most medial common extensor, superior ulnar border	Ulnar base small metacarpal	PIN
EDM	Common extensor origin	Small extensor apparatus	PIN
EDC	Common extensor origin	Digital extensor apparatus	PIN
Deep extensor muscles			
Supinator	Lateral epicondyle, annular ligament, lateral ulnar collateral ligament, crista supinatoris	Anterior proximal radius	PIN
APL	Radius	Thumb metacarpal, base, trapezium, thenar muscle (varies)	PIN
EPB	Interosseous membrane ± radius	Varies: thumb proximal phalanx, extensor hood	PIN
EPL	Ulna	Thumb distal phalanx	PIN
EIP	Ulna + interosseous membrane	Index extensor apparatus	PIN

FOREARM (Figs. 3.2-1 and 3.2-2)

Extensor Carpi Radialis Brevis

- Often, no definite separation between ECRB and extensor digitorum communis (EDC) tendon origin at the osseotendinous junction

Anconeus

- Action: elbow extensor + forearm pronator
- The arterial supply to the anconeus is based on three pedicles: (1) recurrent posterior interosseous artery; (2) medial collateral artery; (3) posterior branch of the radial collateral artery.
- Nerve to the anconeus–branch of radial nerve that arises in the midbrachium and runs within the substance of the medial head of the triceps muscle

■ *Clinical Correlate:* The anconeus muscle may be used as a rotational flap for local tissue reconstruction. Typically, the medial collateral artery is used as a vascular pedicle.

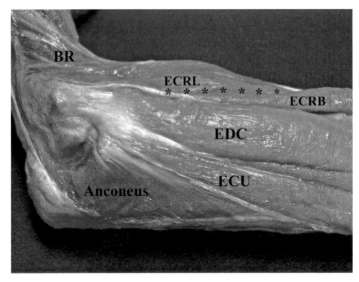

FIGURE 3.2-1 Lateral view of the right elbow demonstrating the extensor origin. The mobile wad of three originates from the lateral supracondylar ridge of the humerus and includes the brachioradialis *(BR)* and the extensor carpi radialis longus and brevis *(ECRL* and *ECRB)*. The ECRB is deep to the ECRL and common extensors at the elbow and is not visualized proximally. The ECRB is identified from the ECRL by markers *(**)*. The extensor digitorum communis *(EDC)* and extensor carpi ulnaris *(ECU)* originate at the lateral epicondyle/condyle as part of the common extensor origin. The sail-shaped **anconeus** muscle originates at the lateral epicondyle and has a broad insertion into the posterior proximal ulna. The surgical interval between the anconeus and the ECU is known as the Kocher interval.

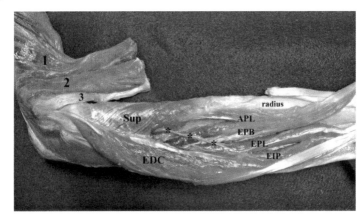

FIGURE 3.2-2 The extensor forearm **(right)** following resection of the central portion of the mobile wad and exposure of the deep muscular structures of the dorsal forearm by ulnar reflection of the extensor digitorum communis *(EDC)* muscle. The brachioradialis *(1)*, extensor carpi radialis longus *(2)*, and extensor carpi radialis brevis *(3)* muscles originate at the lateral supracondylar ridge of the distal humerus. The ECRL has been elevated to expose the deeper tendinous origin of the ECRB. The supinator *(Sup)* origin includes a superficial head (lateral epicondyle and lateral ulnar collateral ligament) and a deep head (crista supinatoris of ulna and annular ligament); the supinator inserts into the anterior surface of the proximal **radius.** The posterior interosseous nerve *(**)* courses distally between the superficial and deep heads of the supinator before arborizing to send three motor branches to the ECU, EDM, and EDC, and two motor branches to the APL, EPL, EPB, and EIP. The abductor pollicis longus *(APL)* origin is identified at the dorsal radius, ulna, and interosseous membrane. The extensor pollicis brevis *(EPB)* that joins the APL within the first dorsal extensor compartment at the wrist originates from the dorsal surfaces of the radius and interosseous membrane. The extensor pollicis longus *(EPL)* and extensor indicis proprius *(EIP)* originate from the dorsal aspect of the interosseous membrane and dorsal mid-diaphyseal ulna.

Supinator

- The arcade of Frohse, approximately 5 cm distal to the lateral epicondyle, is membranous in approximately 68%, and tendinous in 32%, although a tendinous arcade has been described in as high as 87%.
- Innervated by one to six branches from the PIN

WRIST (Figs. 3.2-3 to 3.2-6)

- The extensor retinaculum is a 2-cm-wide fibrous band that acts as a pulley to restrict tendon bowstringing and to maximize biomechanical efficiency for digital and wrist extension.
- The extensor retinaculum attaches radially at the distal radius and has a complex attachment ulnarly into the pisiform, flexor carpi ulnaris, small metacarpal, pisometacarpal ligament, and the abductor digiti minimi muscle.
- At the wrist, there are six synovial, dorsal fibro-osseous compartments beneath the extensor retinaculum.

FIRST EXTENSOR COMPARTMENT (APL + EPB) (Figs. 3.2-7 and 3.2-8)

- APL is palmar and radial to EPB.
- APL may have one or multiple slips; most common: two slips (~70%).
- APL accessory insertion into opponens ± APB ± trapezium
- Typically, EPB has one slip; may be within own subcompartment (~30%).
- First dorsal extensor tendons cross those of the second compartment ~7 cm proximal to the wrist crease.

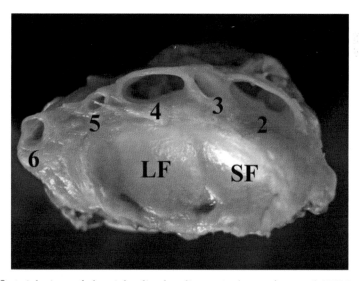

FIGURE 3.2-3 Axial view of the right distal radius articular surface and TFCC after soft tissue removal. The extensor retinaculum and the vertical septa have been preserved to appreciate the second to sixth extensor compartments at the level of the wrist. Note that the fifth extensor compartment (extensor digitorum minimi/quinti) overlies the distal radioulnar joint (*SF*, scaphoid fossa; *LF*, lunate fossa; *2*, second extensor compartment containing ECRL and ECRB; *3*, third extensor compartment with EPL; *4*, fourth extensor compartment with EDC and EIP; *5*, fifth extensor compartment with EDM/EDQ; *6*, sixth extensor compartment with ECU).

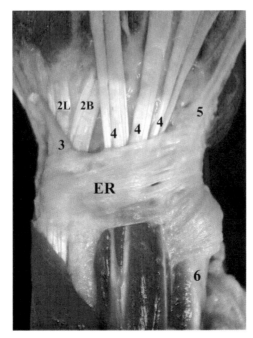

FIGURE 3.2-4 Dorsal view of the right distal forearm and wrist. The muscle of the first dorsal extensor compartment is seen crossing the extensor carpi radialis brevis *(2B)* and longus *(2A)* tendons from ulnar to radial in the distal forearm. The extensor retinaculum serves as the roof for the underlying extensor compartments: *(1)* tendons not visualized, abductor pollicis longus (APL) and extensor pollicis brevis (EPB); *(2)* extensor carpi radialis longus (ECRL) **(2A)** and extensor carpi radialis brevis (ECRB) **(2B)**; *(3)* extensor pollicis longus (EPL); *(4)* extensor digitorum communis (EDC) and extensor indicis proprius (EIP)—EIP not seen, located deep and ulnar to EDC to index finger; *(5)* extensor digiti minimi (EDM)—also referred to as the extensor digitorum quinti (EDQ); *(6)* extensor carpi ulnaris (ECU)—visualized proximal to the ER.

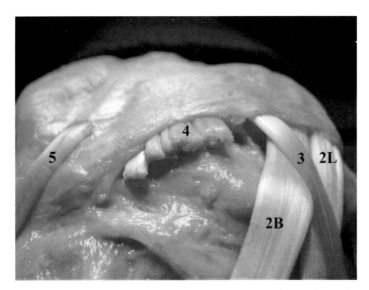

FIGURE 3.2-5 End-on view of the extensor compartments at the level of the distal extensor retinaculum (left wrist) with the wrist held in flexion. The extensor pollicis longus tendon *(3)* crosses the extensor carpi radialis brevis *(2B)* and longus *(2L)* as it courses distal to Lister's tubercle at the distal radius. The extensor digitorum communis and extensor indicis proprius (EIP) tendons make up the fourth dorsal compartment *(4)*; typically, the EIP muscle belly extends most distally. The extensor digiti minimi *(5)* is located dorsal to the distal radioulnar joint (DRUJ).

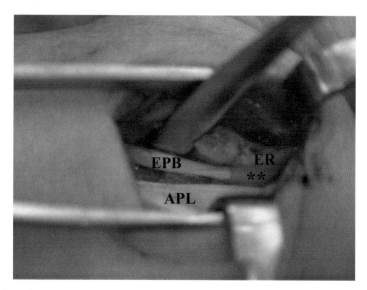

FIGURE 3.2-6 Midsagittal aspect of the left radial wrist (**top** of figure is dorsal), demonstrating an exposure of the first dorsal extensor compartment during a de Quervain's release. The extensor retinaculum *(ER)* has been incised to reveal the extensor pollicis brevis *(EPB)* tendon that is dorsal to the abductor pollicis longus *(APL)* tendon. In this case, it is important to note that as the EPB courses distally within the first extensor compartment, it enters into its own subcompartment *(**)* that needs to be decompressed, also.

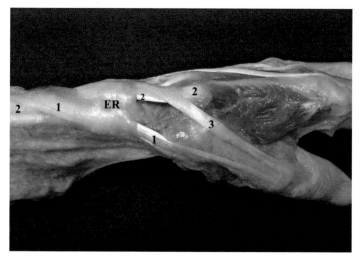

FIGURE 3.2-7 Lateral view of the pronated left forearm and wrist demonstrating the first *(1)*, second *(2)*, and third *(3)* dorsal extensor compartments of the wrist. The compartmentalization of the extensor tendons is created by osteofascial compartments, including the extensor retinaculum *(ER)* that spans from the radius to the ulna. The first compartment *(1)*, which contains the abductor pollicis longus (APL) and extensor pollicis brevis (EPB) tendons, is identified as it runs superficial to the second compartment *(2)*, from ulnar to radial, coursing distally to the thumb. In the third dorsal compartment *(3)*, the extensor pollicis longus (EPL) passes superficial to the ECRL and ECRB *(2)*.

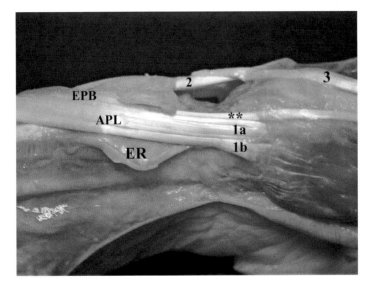

FIGURE 3.2-8 Close-up view of the first dorsal extensor compartment at the radial wrist following division of the extensor retinaculum *(ER)*. The multiple tendon slips of the abductor pollicis longus *(APL)* are located volar and radial to the single tendon of the extensor pollicis brevis *(EPB **)*. The APL is seen here as it inserts into the base of the thumb metacarpal *(1a)* and into the fascia overlying the thenar musculature *(1b)*. The EPB may or may not be subcompartmentalized within the first compartment. The second *(2)* and third *(3)* extensor compartments are identified.

■ *Clinical Correlate:* de Quervain's stenosing tenovaginitis/tenosynovitis involves the tendons of the first dorsal compartment. A separate compartment, or subcompartment, containing the EPB tendon may be found during surgical treatment.

SECOND EXTENSOR COMPARTMENT (ECRL + ECRB)

■ *Clinical Correlate:* Pain at the site of the first extensor compartment as it passes dorsal to the second extensor compartment is referred to as "**intersection syndrome**." Patients may have locally associated swelling and crepitance. Palpation of this area has been said to produce a sensation akin to "footprints on freshly packed snow."
■ *Clinically Relevant Anatomical Variation:* The extensor carpi radialis indicis may be found in up to 10%—it arises between the ECRB and ECRL.

THIRD EXTENSOR COMPARTMENT (EPL) (Fig. 3.2-9)

• The EPL originates on the ulna and angles 45° in the radial direction as it courses distal to Lister's tubercle.
• The EPL serves to extend and retropulse the thumb (i.e., lift the thumb off of a flat surface when the palm is placed flat against the surface) and to adduct the thumb, based on its force vector.

FOURTH EXTENSOR COMPARTMENT (EDC + EIP)

• EIP origin is deep to EDC; its muscle belly extends more distally than the other extensors.
• EIP is located ulnar to the index EDC in most cases.

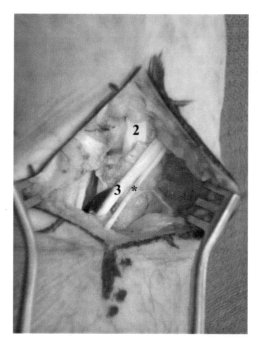

FIGURE 3.2-9 An example of one of the many extensor tendon anomalies in this dorsal exposure of a left wrist. The extensor pollicis longus *(3)* has been exposed within the third extensor compartment, prior to coursing around Lister's tubercle and heading radially toward the thumb, superficial to the second extensor compartment *(2)*. An anomalous, accessory EPL tendon *(*)* is noted in its own subcompartment, superficial to the EPL proper.

- Typically, the long and ring fingers are extended by a single EDC tendon.
- Most commonly, there are two EDM tendons and no EDC to the small finger (~55%). The next most common variant is one EDM + one EDC to the small finger.
- Over the hand, the EDC tendons are interconnected by a series of fascial structures called **juncture tendinae**. The juncture tendinae become more substantial ulnarly.

■ *Clinically Relevant Anatomical Variation:* The extensor digitorum brevis manus (EDBM) may present as a dorsal wrist mass, and should be considered in the differential diagnosis of a dorsal wrist mass. The EDBM (incidence 1% to 3%) originates from the dorsal wrist capsule within the fourth dorsal extensor compartment and has a variable insertion, including to the extensor hood of the index or long fingers.

FIFTH EXTENSOR COMPARTMENT (EDM)

- Fibrous compartment overlies DRUJ

SIXTH EXTENSOR COMPARTMENT (ECU) (Fig. 3.2-10)

- Stabilized by the extensor retinaculum and a subcompartment, the **linea jugata**. Failure may lead to ECU subluxation.

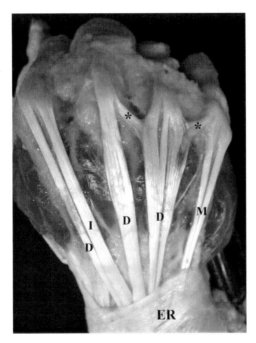

FIGURE 3.2-10 Dorsal view of the right hand demonstrating the most common variation of the extrinsic extensor anatomy distal to the extensor retinaculum *(ER)*. In this example, there are tendon slips to the index, long, and ring fingers from the extensor digitorum communis *(D)*; however, the small finger has no EDC but has two tendon slips from the extensor digiti minimi *(M)*. The extensor indicis proprius *(I)* tendon is ulnar to the EDC tendon; this is similar to the ulnar orientation of the EDM tendon when the EDC contributes a tendon to the small finger. The juncturae tendinae are noted between the long–ring and ring–small extrinsic tendons *(*)*.

RECOMMENDED READING

Albright J, Linburg R. Common variations of the radial wrist extensors. *J Hand Surg.* 1978;3:134–138.

Bearn JG. The history of the ideas on the function of the biceps brachii muscle as a supinator. *Med Hist.* 1963;7:32–42.

Branovacki G, Hanson M, Cash R, et al. The innervations pattern of the radial nerve at the elbow and in the forearm. *J Hand Surg Br.* 1998;23:167–169.

Briggs CA, Elliott BG. Lateral epicondylitis: a review of structures associated with tennis elbow. *Anat Clin.* 1985;7:149–153.

Dahners LE, Wood FM. Anconeus epitrochlearis, a rare cause of cubital tunnel syndrome: a case report. *J Hand Surg.* 1984;9A:579–580.

Debouck C, Rooze M. The arcade of Frohse: an anatomic study. *Surg Radiol Anat.* 1995;17:245–248.

el-Badawi MG, Butt MM, al-Zuhair AG, et al. Extensor tendons of the fingers: arrangement and variations. *Clin Anat.* 1995;8:391–398.

Freehafer AA, Peckham PH, Keith MW, et al. The brachioradialis: anatomy, properties, and value for tendon transfer in the tetraplegic. *J Hand Surg.* 1988;13A:99–104.

Gonzalez MH, Gray T, Ortinau E, et al. The extensor tendons to the little finger: an anatomic study. *J Hand Surg.* 1995;20:844–847.

Gonzalez MH, Sohlberg R, Brown A, et al. The first dorsal compartment: an anatomic study. *J Hand Surg.* 1995;20:657–660.

Gonzalez MH, Weinzweig N, Kay T, et al. Anatomy of the extensor tendons to the index finger. *J Hand Surg.* 1996;21A:988–991.

Greenbaum B, Itamura J, Vangsness CT, et al. Extensor carpi radialis brevis. An anatomical analysis of its origin. *J Bone Joint Surg Br.* 1999;81:926–929.

Grundberg AB, Reagan DS. Pathologic anatomy of the forearm: intersection syndrome. *J Hand Surg.* 1985;10:299–302.

Guillot M, Escande G, Chazal J, et al. The anconeus muscle. Anatomical and electromyographic study. *Bull Assoc Anat (Nancy).* 1984;68:337–343.

Hirai Y, Yoshida K, Yamanaka K, et al. An anatomic study of the extensor tendons of the human hand. *J Hand Surg.* 2001;26A:1009–1015.

Jackson WT, Viegas SF, Coon TM, et al. Anatomical variations in the first extensor compartment of the wrist. A clinical and anatomical study. *J Bone Joint Surg.* 1986;68A:923–926.

Leslie BM, Ericson WB, Morehead JR. Incidence of a septum within the first dorsal compartment of the wrist. *J Hand Surg.* 1990;15A:88–91.

Ozturk A, Kutlu C, Taskara N, et al. Anatomic and morphometric study of the arcade of Frohse in cadavers. *Surg Radiol Anat.* 2005;27:171–175.

Pevny T, Rayan GM, Egle D. Ligamentous and tendinous support of the pisiform, anatomic and biomechanical study. *J Hand Surg.* 1995;20A:299–304.

Rodriguez-Niedenfuhr M, Vazquez T, Golano P, et al. Extensor digitorum brevis manus: anatomical, radiological and clinical relevance. A review. *Clin Anat.* 2002;15:286–292.

Schmidt CC, Kohut GN, Greenberg JA, et al. The anconeus muscle flap: its anatomy and clinical application. *J Hand Surg.* 1999;24A:359–369.

Spinner M. The arcade of Frohse and its relationship to posterior interosseous nerve paralysis. *J Bone Joint Surg.* 1968;50B:809–812.

Spinner M, Kaplan EB. Extensor carpi ulnaris. Its relationship to the stability of the distal radio-ulnar joint. *Clin Orthop Relat Res.* 1970;68:124–129.

Taleisnik J, Gelberman RH, Miller BW, et al. The extensor retinaculum of the wrist. *J Hand Surg.* 1984;9:495–701.

Tan ST, Smith PJ. Anomalous extensor muscles of the hand: a review. *J Hand Surg.* 1999;24A:449–455.

Thomas SJ, Yakin DE, Parry BR, et al. The anatomical relationship between the posterior interosseous nerve and the supinator muscle. *J Hand Surg.* 2000;25A:936–941.

von Oudenaarde E. Structure and function of the abductor pollicis longus muscle. *J Anat.* 1991;174:221–227.

von Schroeder HP, Botte MJ. The extensor medii proprius and anomalous extensor tendons to the long finger. *J Hand Surg.* 1991;16A:1141–1145.

von Schroeder HP, Botte MJ. Anatomy of the extensor tendons of the fingers: variations and multiplicity. *J Hand Surg.* 1995;20:27–34.

von Schroeder HP, Botte MJ, Gellman H. Anatomy of the juncturae tendinum of the hand. *J Hand Surg.* 1990;15A:595–602.

Wehbe MA. Anatomy of the extensor mechanism of the hand and wrist. *Hand Clin.* 1995;11:361–366.

Witt J, Pess G, Gelberman RH. Treatment of de Quervain tenosynovitis. *J Bone Joint Surg.* 1991;73:219–222.

3.3   Antecubital Fossa and Volar Forearm

ANTECUBITAL FOSSA (Figs. 3.3-1 to 3.3-3)

- **Borders**
  - Roof: lacertus fibrosus
  - Floor: brachialis muscle; supinator muscle laterally
  - Ulnar border: pronator teres muscle
  - Radial border: brachioradialis muscle
  - Proximal border: interepicondylar line of the distal humerus

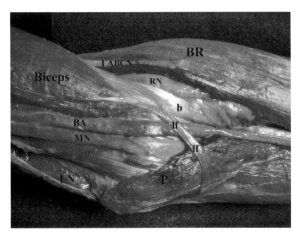

FIGURE 3.3-1 View of the antecubital fossa of the left elbow. Neurovascular and muscular relationships are well defined in this example. The lateral antebrachial cutaneous nerve *(LABCN >)* that provides sensation to the ulnar forearm descends along the lateral border of the **biceps** brachii muscle, piercing the brachial fascia at approximately the level of the interepicondylar line of the elbow. The radial nerve *(RN)* courses deep within the biceps–brachioradialis *(BR)* muscular interval. The biceps, which is superficial to the underlying brachialis muscle, remains lateral to the median nerve *(MN)* and the brachial artery *(BA)*; the median nerve remains medial to the brachial artery as they descend into the forearm deep to the lacertus fibrosus *(lf)* or bicipital aponeurosis, a fascial division of the biceps muscle that courses medially and superficial to the flexor–pronator muscular origin to insert into the antebrachial fascia. The pronator teres muscle *(P)* originates as a superficial head (medial supracondylar ridge and medial epicondyle) and deep head (medial border of coronoid, distal to the sublime tubercle). The biceps tendon proper *(b)* inserts into the radial tuberosity of the proximal radius. The ulnar nerve *(UN)* is visualized through a window of excised medial intermuscular septum; the ulnar nerve remains in the posterior compartment of the brachium prior to entering the cubital tunnel at the elbow.

- **Structures on roof**
  - **Medial antebrachial cutaneous nerve (MABCN)**
    - Anterior branch passes 2 to 3 cm lateral to medial epicondyle.
    - Posterior branch crosses ulnar nerve anywhere from 6 cm proximal to 4 cm distal to medial epicondyle.

■ *Clinical Correlate:* Injury to the MABCN during surgical dissection, such as for operative treatment of cubital tunnel syndrome, may place the patient at risk for developing chronic regional pain syndrome (CRPS 2).

  - **Median basilic vein**
  - **Lateral antebrachial cutaneous nerve (LABCN)**
    - Terminal portion of musculocutaneous nerve
    - Becomes subcutaneous after passing between the biceps brachii and the brachialis muscular interval
    - Provides independent sensation to a 1- to 2-in.-wide patch of skin on the volar lateral distal forearm and thumb
  - **Cephalic vein**
- **Contents of the antecubital fossa** (medial to lateral)
  - **Anterior ulnar recurrent artery**

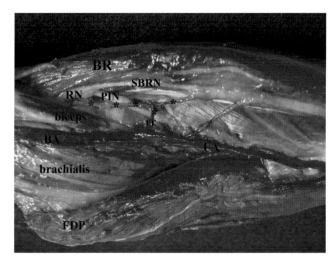

FIGURE 3.3-2 View of the antecubital fossa of the left elbow following resection of the flexor digitorum superficialis and pronator teres muscles and the median nerve. The brachial artery *(BA)* that lies superficial to the **brachialis** muscle and medial to the **biceps** brachii muscle commonly divides into the radial artery and ulnar artery *(UA)*, although many variations of this arterial branching have been described. The radial recurrent artery (*rr* and ******), which has variable origins also, is identified branching from the brachial artery proximal to the ulnar artery. It is observed here in proximity to the radial nerve *(RN)* and its terminal branches, the superficial branch of the radial nerve *(SBRN)* and the posterior interosseous nerve *(PIN)*. The recurrent radial artery is an important source of vascular supply to the brachioradialis muscle *(BR)*. The anatomical course of the ulnar artery may be appreciated here; the ulnar artery *(UA)* lies deep to the pronator teres muscle and courses distally and ulnarward on the volar surface of the flexor digitorum profundus *(FDP)* muscle (deep flexor).

- **Median nerve**
  - Lies medial to the brachial artery and superficial to the brachialis muscle
  - Typically enters forearm between the humeral and ulnar heads of the pronator teres
- **Brachial artery**
  - Lies lateral to the medial nerve superficial to the brachialis muscle
  - Bifurcates into radial and ulnar arteries
- **Biceps tendon**
  - Inserts onto the bicipital tuberosity (proximal radius)
  - Lacertus fibrosus is the fibrous extension of the biceps tendon that fans medially and inserts into the fascia of pronator teres. It provides additional insertion of biceps tendon.
- **Radial recurrent artery**
- **Radial nerve**
  - Becomes anterior in the arm approximately 10 cm proximal to the lateral epicondyle
  - Runs directly over the radiocapitellar joint
  - Divides into the SBRN and PIN

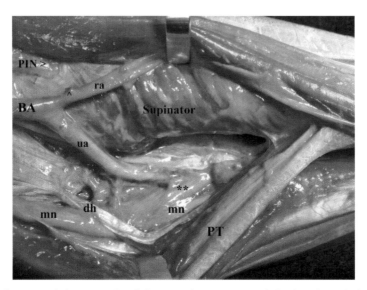

FIGURE 3.3-3 View of the antecubital fossa with retraction of the brachioradialis muscle (top) and pronator teres muscle *(PT)*. Note that the median nerve has been displaced medially, away from the brachial artery with this retraction. The posterior interosseous nerve *(PIN >)* is identified as it enters the supinator muscle in the proximal forearm. The brachial artery *(BA)* bifurcates into the radial artery *(ra)* and ulnar artery *(ua)*. In this example, the recurrent radial artery *(cut)* originates from the radial artery *(^)*. The ulnar artery is traced distally, deep to the pronator teres and median nerve. The median nerve *(mn)* courses between the deep *(dh)* and superficial heads of the pronator teres *(PT)* muscle. The anterior interosseous nerve *(**)* branches from the median nerve to supply motor innervation to the flexor digitorum profundus (index and long), the flexor pollicis longus, and the pronator quadratus muscles. The median nerve *(mn)* continues distally in the FDS–FDP interval, commonly contained within the FDS epimysium, although it has been described to run within the FDS muscle substance.

VOLAR FOREARM (Fig. 3.3-4)

• Musculature may be considered in two groups:

Muscle	Origin	Insertion	Innervation
Superficial layer (all cross elbow joint)			
Pronator teres	*Superficial head:* distal 1 cm of supracondylar ridge + medial epicondyle	Midlateral radius	Median nerve
	Deep head: medial coronoid	Distal to sublime tubercle	
FCR	Medial epicondyle	Index + long metacarpal bases	Median nerve
PL	Medial epicondyle	Palmar aponeurosis	Median nerve

(continued)

Muscle	Origin	Insertion	Innervation
FDS	Medial epicondyle, sublime tubercle, anterior radius	Base of P2 (fingers)	Median nerve
FCU	*Humeral head:* medial epicondyle *Ulnar head:* posteromedial ulna	Pisiform, pisohamate-ligament, Pisometacarpal ligament	Ulnar nerve
Deep layer (do not cross elbow joint) (Fig. 3.3-5)			
FDP	Anterior + medial ulna, interosseous membrane	Base of P3 (fingers)	AIN and ulnar nerve
FPL	Anterior radius, interosseous membrane	Base of thumb P2	AIN
Pronator quadratus	Distal ulna	Volar radius	AIN

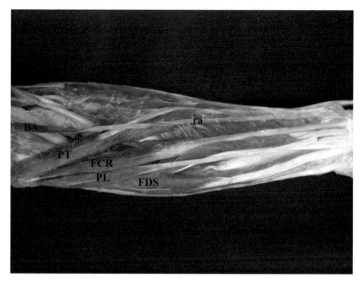

FIGURE 3.3-4 The volar forearm demonstrates the orientation and relationships of the superficial musculature. The pronator teres *(PT)*, flexor carpi radialis *(FCR)*, and palmaris longus course obliquely and are superficial to the common origin of the flexor digitorum superficialis *(FDS)*. The vascular relationships are demonstrated as the brachial artery *(BA)* divides into the radial artery *(ra)* and the ulnar artery *(u)*; the radial artery remains superficial to the pronator teres and the flexor musculature while the ulnar artery descends deep to the pronator teres muscle.

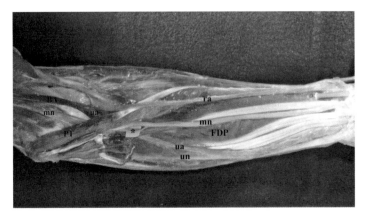

FIGURE 3.3-5 Similar dissection of the volar forearm as Figure 3.3-4; however, the superficial flexors (FCR, palmaris, FDS) have been removed. The course of the ulnar artery *(ua)*, deep to the pronator teres *(PT)* and deep to the median nerve *(mn)*, is followed distally as it heads medially over the volar surface of the flexor digitorum profundus muscle *(FDP)* to meet the ulnar nerve in the midforearm. The ulnar artery remains radial/lateral to the ulnar nerve throughout the forearm. The anterior interosseous nerve is identified *(*)*. Note the dorsal insertion of the pronator teres along the mid-diaphysis of the radius.

VOLAR FOREARM (Figs. 3.3-6 to 3.3-8)

Pronator Teres

- Deep (ulnar) head of pronator teres may be absent in ~6%.
- Ligament of Struthers, when present, forms an accessory humeral origin.
- Deep head of the pronator teres separates the **ulnar artery** (deep to the deep muscular head) **from the median nerve** (superficial to deep head).

Flexor Carpi Radialis

- Musculotendinous junction begins 12 to 17 cm proximal to volar wrist crease
- The tendon enters a fibro-osseous tunnel at the proximal aspect of the trapezium and courses dorsally to insert into (1) trapezial tuberosity (small tendinous slip); (2) index metacarpal base (80% of substance); and (3) long metacarpal base (20% of substance).
- The tendon is separated from the carpal tunnel by a fibrous septum; the distal portion of the septum is a pivot point around which the FPL courses toward the thumb.

Palmaris Longus

- **Palmaris longus** may be absent in ~15% (unilateral) and 7% (bilateral).

Flexor Digitorium Superficialis and Profundus

- The two FDS heads (ulnohumeral and radial) form a broad, arching origin of the FDS that may be primarily tendinous (75%) or muscular (25%) and may be a site of median nerve compression.
- The median nerve courses distally between the FDS and FDP: commonly within the FDS epimysium, and occasionally within the FDS substance.

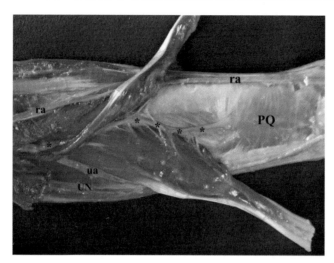

FIGURE 3.3-6 Deep flexor forearm after resection of the FCR and FDS muscles. The flexor digitorum profundus (FDP) muscle bellies have been elevated (index—**top**; long/ring/small—**bottom**) revealing the anatomical course of the anterior interosseous nerve *(**)*, through the FDP muscle substance and dorsal to the pronator quadratus *(PQ)* muscle at the distal forearm. Branches of the AIN to the FDP muscle are appreciated. The relationship of the radial artery *(ra)* to the superficial flexors *(cut)* and the relationship of the ulnar nerve *(UN)* and artery *(ua)* are demonstrated.

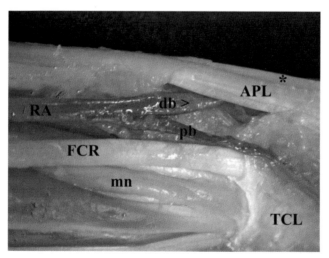

FIGURE 3.3-7 Relationship of the radial artery *(RA)* and its deep branch *(db >)* and palmar branch *(pb)* to the structures of the volar and radial wrist. The radial artery is immediately volar and ulnar to the brachioradialis tendon and to the first dorsal extensor compartment tendons *(APL,* abductor pollicis longus; **,* extensor pollicis brevis). Note the intimate relationship of the palmar branch of the radial artery *(pb)* to the volar surface of the distal flexor carpi radialis tendon *(FCR)*. The deep branch of the radial artery *(db)* passes deep to the first dorsal extensor compartment tendons at the level of the radial snuffbox of the wrist. The median nerve *(mn)* is noted ulnar to the **FCR** tendon and radial to the FDS muscle before entering the carpal tunnel at the leading edge of the transverse carpal ligament *(TCL)*.

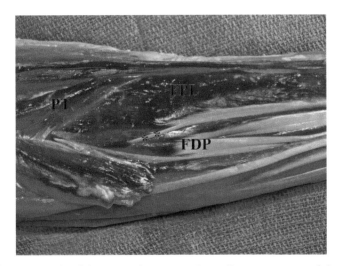

FIGURE 3.3-8 An example of the anomalous musculotendinous anatomy of the forearm. The tendinous interconnection *(**)* between the flexor digitorum profundus *(FDP)* to the index finger and the flexor pollicis longus *(FPL)* has been described (Linburg–Comstock interconnection) and may be present unilaterally in 25% to 30% and bilaterally in 5% to 15%. *PT*, pronator teres.

- Independent active FDS function to the small finger **is absent in up to 75%**.
- At the wrist, the long and ring finger FDS tendons are **volar** to those of the index and small fingers.

Flexor Carpi Ulnaris

- The flexor carpi ulnaris is the most ulnar tendon at the volar wrist, with muscle fibers extending distally to the level of its insertion.

Pronator Quadratus

- A distinct muscular compartment within the volar forearm

■ *Clinical Correlate:* The pronator quadratus muscle may be an independent compartment within the volar forearm, at risk for elevated tissue pressures and compartment syndrome.

■ *Clinical Relevant Anatomical Variants:*
1. The anconeus epitrochlearis muscle (incidence 11%) overlying the cubital tunnel at the elbow may be a cause of compressive neuropathy of the ulnar nerve at the elbow (cubital tunnel syndrome). The muscle originates at the medial epicondyle and inserts into the olecranon.
2. The flexor pollicis longus (FPL) may have an accessory head, originating from the proximal ulna or medial epicondyle (Gantzer's muscle).
3. A tendinous interconnection (Linburg–Comstock) between the index FDP and FPL may be present in the forearm (25% to 30% unilateral; 5% to 15% bilateral), resulting in an interdependence of tendon excursion between the two tendons.

4. The palmar profundus muscle arises from the radius at the proximal FPL origin and inserts into the transverse carpal ligament.
5. The flexor carpi radialis brevis muscle originates from the radius at the proximal FPL origin and merges with the FCR in the distal forearm.

RECOMMENDED READING

al-Qattan MM. Gantzer's muscle. An anatomical study of the accessory head of the flexor pollicis longus muscle. *J Hand Surg Br.* 1996;21:269–270.

Armenta E, Fisher J. Anatomy of the flexor pollicis longus vinculum system. *J Hand Surg.* 1984;9A:210–212.

Azar CA, Culver JE, Fleegler EJ. Blood supply of the flexor pollicis longus tendon. *J Hand Surg.* 1983;8A:471–475.

Beaton LE, Anson BJ. The relation of the median nerve to the pronator teres muscle. *Anat Rec.* 1939;75:23–26.

Bishop AT, Gabel G, Carmichael SW. Flexor carpi radialis tendinitis. Part I: operative anatomy. *J Bone Joint Surg.* 1994;76A:1009–1014.

Bourne MH, Wood MB, Carmichael SW. Locating the lateral antebrachial cutaneous nerve. *J Hand Surg.* 1987;12A:697–699.

Grechenig W, Clement H, Egner S, et al. Musculotendinous junction of the flexor carpi ulnaris muscle. An anatomical study. *Surg Radiol Anat.* 2000;22:255–260.

Hergenroeder PT, Gelberman RH, Akeson WH. The vascularity of the flexor pollicis longus tendon. *Clin Orthop Relat Res.* 1982;162:298–303.

Linburg RM, Comstock BE. Anomalous tendon slips from the flexor pollicis longus to the flexor digitorum profundus. *J Hand Surg.* 1979;4:79–83.

Nebot-Cegarra J, Perez-Berruezo J, Reina de la Torre F. Variations of the pronator teres muscle: predispositional role to median nerve entrapment. *Arch Anat Histol Embryol.* 1991;74:35–45.

Nigro RO. Anatomy of the flexor retinaculum of the wrist and the flexor carpi radialis tunnel. *Hand Clin.* 2001;17:61–64.

Reimann AF, Daseler EH, Anson BJ, et al. The palmaris longus muscle and tendon: a study of 1600 extremities. *Anat Rec.* 1944;89:495.

Schmidt HM. Clinical anatomy of the m. flexor carpi radialis tendon sheath. *Acta Morphol Neerl Scand.* 1987;25:17–28.

Sotereanos DG, McCarthy DM, Towers JD, et al. The pronator quadratus: a distinct forearm space? *J Hand Surg.* 1995;20A:496–499.

Tubbs RS, Marshall T, Loukas M, et al. The sublime bridge: anatomy and implications in median nerve entrapment. *J Neurosurg.* 2009.

3.4   Cross-Sectional Anatomy of the Forearm

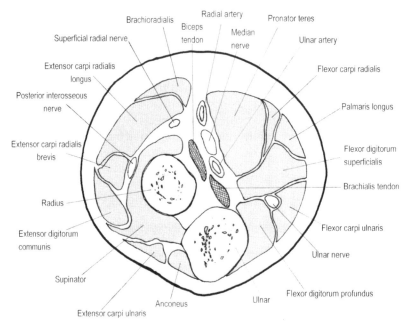

FIGURE 3.4-1 Cross-section illustration of the forearm, proximal to the biceps tuberosity.

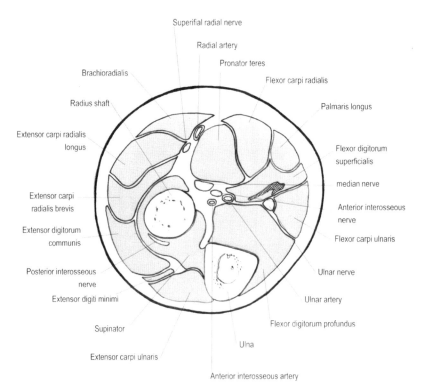

FIGURE 3.4-2 Cross-section illustration of the forearm at the origin of the anterior interosseous nerve.

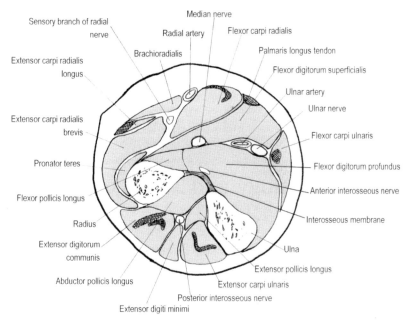

FIGURE 3.4-3 Cross-section illustration of the middle 1/3 forearm.

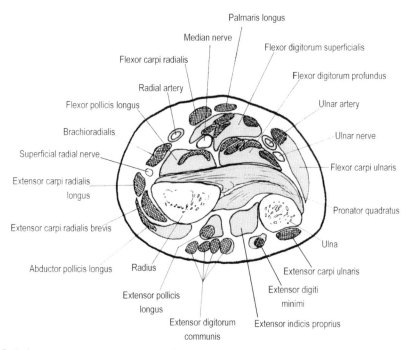

FIGURE 3.4-4 Cross-section illustration of the distal forearm.

4 Elbow

4.1 Osteology and Joints of the Elbow (Figs. 4.1-1 to 4.1-6)

- Complex articulations between the distal humerus, the proximal radius, and the proximal ulna.

DISTAL HUMERUS

- The distal humerus consists of two condyles (medial and lateral) supported proximally by their respective bony columns that create an arch over a central area comprised of the olecranon fossa (posterior) and the coronoid fossa (anterior).
- The coronoid fossa and the olecranon fossa accommodate the coronoid tip and the olecranon tip during flexion and extension of the elbow, respectively.
- The distal humerus articular surface is angled 30° anteriorly, with 5° to 7° internal rotation, and 6° to 7° valgus alignment.
- The articular surfaces of the distal humerus:
  - Medial: **trochlea**
    - Articulates with semilunar notch of proximal ulna
    - Medial aspect is larger than its lateral counterpart and it projects more distally
    - Trochlear sulcus runs from anterolateral to posteromedial
  - Lateral: **capitellum**
    - Articulates with radial head
    - Hemispherical, projecting anteriorly and inferiorly
    - Articular surface does not extend posterior to the coronal plane of the anterior humerus
- The **medial epicondyle** is a bony prominence projecting medially from the medial condyle. It serves as the attachment for the medial collateral ligament and the flexor–pronator musculotendinous origins.
- The **lateral epicondyle** that projects laterally from the lateral condyle, just proximal to the capitellum, is the attachment site of the lateral ulnar collateral ligament and the extensor–supinator musculotendinous origins.

PROXIMAL ULNA

- **Greater sigmoid notch** (where ulna articulates with the trochlea)
  - Alignment: 30° posterior angulation, 4° valgus alignment
  - 190° arc
  - Typically, divided into anterior and posterior articular surfaces by a transversely oriented area of nonarticular cartilage

- **Lesser sigmoid notch** (proximal radioulnar joint)
  - 60° to 80° arc
  - Located slightly distal to the lateral margin of the coronoid
- **Crista supinatoris**: insertion site of the lateral ulnar collateral ligament
- **Sublime tubercle**: insertion site of the anterior band of the ulnar collateral ligament
- **Coronoid process**: the brachialis tendon inserts into its anterior cortical surface
- **Olecranon process**: the triceps inserts into its proximal aspect

PROXIMAL RADIUS

- Disc-shaped head with central depression to accommodate the capitellum.
- The radial head has 240° articulation with the ulna at the lesser sigmoid notch.
- The radial neck angles ~15° from the long axis of the radial diaphysis.
- The **radial tuberosity** defines the distal margin of the radial neck and is comprised of two parts:
  - Anterior: covered by bicipitoradial bursa
  - Posterior: biceps tendon insertion site
- The radial tuberosity is located posteriorly with the forearm in maximal pronation.

ELBOW JOINT

- A complex joint consisting of three articulations:
  - **Ulnohumeral joint**
    - Hinge joint (ginglymus)
  - **Radiocapitellar joint**
    - Rotational joint
  - **Proximal radioulnar joint**
    - Rotational joint
- Carrying angle: male: 11° to 14° valgus; female: 13° to 16° valgus
- Elbow axis of rotation is **from the lateral epicondyle through the anterior–inferior margin of the medial epicondyle**.
- Joint volume: average capacity of 27 mL
- The **joint capsule** inserts proximal to the coronoid and radial fossa anteriorly and proximal to the olecranon fossa posteriorly. Distally, the capsule attaches distal to the tip of the coronoid process anteriorly, and along the medial and lateral margins of the sigmoid notch.

■ *Clinical Correlate:* Coronoid tip fractures are evidence of joint instability.

4.2   Ligamentous Anatomy of the Elbow

MEDIAL COLLATERAL LIGAMENT COMPLEX (MCL)

Comprised of three ligamentous bundles:
1. Anterior bundle
2. Posterior bundle
3. Transverse bundle
- **Anterior bundle (anterior medial collateral ligament)**
  - **Origin**: anterior–inferior aspect of the medial epicondyle
  - **Insertion**: sublime tubercle on the medial side of the coronoid

- Subdivided into anterior, posterior, and deep bands
- Anterior bands: taut in extension; posterior bands: taut in flexion
- Dimensions: approximately 5 × 27 mm
- Primary stabilizer of the medial elbow

■ *Clinical Correlate*: May be injured with severe valgus force to the elbow; typically is symptomatic in the throwing athlete after injury.

- **Posterior bundle**
  - **Origin**: anterior–inferior aspect of the medial epicondyle
  - **Insertion**: midportion of medial aspect of semilunar notch
  - Important stabilizer with the elbow in flexion
  - Thickening of posterior capsule, accentuated in elbow flexion
- **Transverse bundle (ligament of Cooper)**
  - Provides minimal stabilizing support to the medial joint

LATERAL COLLATERAL LIGAMENT COMPLEX (LCL)

- Considered a complex of ligaments, rather than individual, discrete ligaments; made up of several components:
  1. Lateral ulnar collateral ligament
  2. Radial collateral ligament
  3. Annular ligament
  4. Accessory lateral collateral ligament
- **Lateral ulnar collateral ligament (LUCL)**
  - **Origin**: lateral epicondyle (central; at isometric point)
  - **Insertion**: tubercle of the supinator crest of the proximal ulna
  - Taut throughout flexion and extension of the elbow
  - **Primary stabilizer of the lateral elbow**
  - Deficient in posterolateral rotational instability of the elbow

■ *Clinical Correlate*: The LUCL is injured in all elbow dislocations. Immobilization with the forearm in pronation and the elbow flexed may maintain a stable reduction, but protected motion should be initiated within 3 weeks of injury to minimize stiffness.

- **Radial collateral ligament (RCL)**
  - **Origin**: lateral epicondyle
  - **Insertion**: annular ligament
  - **Dimensions**: width—8 mm; length—20 mm
- **Annular ligament**
  - **Origin**: anterior margin of lesser sigmoid notch
  - **Insertion**: posterior margin of lesser sigmoid notch
  - Stabilizes proximal radius to ulna
- **Accessory lateral collateral ligament**
  - **Origin**: fibers merge with annular ligament
  - **Insertion**: ulnar fibers inserting into tubercle of supinator crest

OBLIQUE CORD

- Variable presence; thickened fascia overlying deep head of supinator
- **Origin**: lateral margin of tuberosity of proximal ulna
- **Insertion**: radius, just distal to tuberosity

QUADRATE LIGAMENT (LIGAMENT OF DENUCE)

- Thin fibrous tissue superficial to anterior capsule
- **Origin**: inferior margin of annular ligament
- **Insertion**: ulna

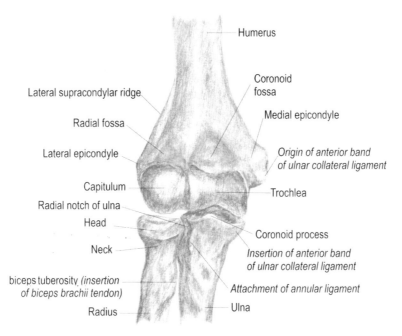

FIGURE 4.1-1 Illustration of the anterior elbow anatomy.

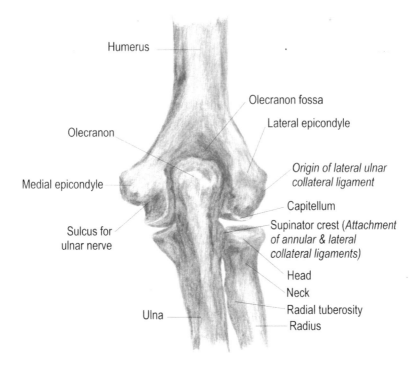

FIGURE 4.1-2 Illustration of the posterior elbow anatomy.

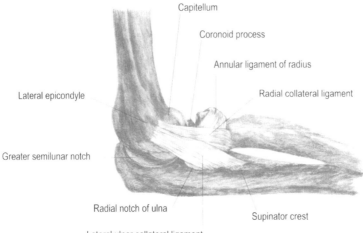

Capitellum

Coronoid process

Annular ligament of radius

Radial collateral ligament

Lateral epicondyle

Greater semilunar notch

Radial notch of ulna

Supinator crest

Lateral ulnar collateral ligament

FIGURE 4.1-3 Illustration of the lateral elbow anatomy.

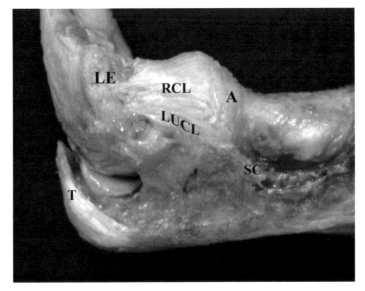

FIGURE 4.1-4 The lateral collateral ligament complex of the elbow originates at the isometric point of elbow rotation at the lateral epicondyle *(LE)*. The lateral ulnar collateral ligament is the primary stabilizer and inserts into the supinator crest *(SC)* of the ulna. The radial collateral ligament *(RCL)* inserts into the annular ligament *(A)*; the annular ligament courses from the anterior to the posterior borders of the lesser sigmoid notch circumferentially about the neck of the proximal radius.

4.3	**Musculotendinous Anatomy of the Elbow**

ANTERIOR ELBOW

Biceps Brachii

- **Origin**: coracoid process (short head) and superior lip of glenoid (long head)
- **Insertion**: distal tendon may have 1 or 2 distinct tendon slips, each a continuation of the long and short heads of the muscle. Short head: inserts slightly distal to radial

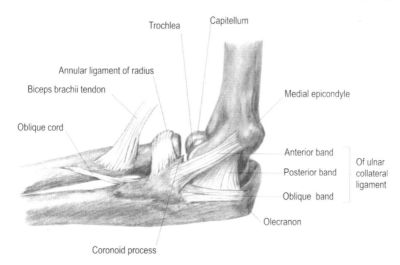

FIGURE 4.1-5 Illustration of the medial elbow anatomy.

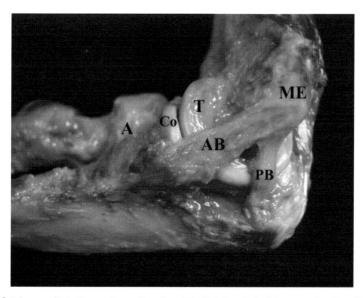

FIGURE 4.1-6 The medial elbow dissection is with distal = left. The anterior bundle of the medial collateral ligament *(AB)* originates at the anterior–inferior aspect of the medial epicondyle *(ME)* and is the primary stabilizer of the medial elbow. It inserts into the sublime tubercle on the medial aspect of the coronoid *(Co)*. The medial collateral ligament is comprised of the anterior bundle *(AB)*, the posterior bundle *(PB)*, and the transverse ligament (not shown). The annular ligament *(A)* and trochlea of the distal humerus *(T)* are identified.

tuberosity and is considered a more powerful elbow flexor. Long head: inserts into radial tuberosity and is advantaged as a supinator of the forearm.

- The **bicipital aponeurosis,** or **lacertus fibrosus,** begins at the distal musculotendinous junction and consists of three layers (superficial, middle, deep) that merge and course distally and ulnarly, superficial to the ulnar flexor musculature. The aponeurosis has distal attachments to (1) ulnar flexor muscles through fascial adhesions;

(2) antebrachial fascia; (3) proximal radial and ulnar aspects of the ulna, after enveloping the forearm flexor muscles.
- **Innervation**: musculocutaneous nerve
- **Function**: (1) forearm supination; (2) elbow flexion
- The **bicipitoradial bursa** surrounds the tendinous insertion of the biceps.

Brachialis

- **Origin**: two heads; larger, superficial head arises from anterolateral aspect of humerus, proximal to the origin of the more anterior deep head.
- **Insertion**: (1) limited fiber attachment to anterior elbow capsule ("articularis cubitus"); (2) superficial head: terminates as circular tendon (28 to 53 mm in length external to muscle) onto the ulnar tuberosity; (3) deep head converges as an aponeurosis to insert medial to the superficial head, attaching to all but the tip of the coronoid process
- **Innervation**: musculocutaneous nerve, except for **inferolateral fibers of the deep head which are innervated by the radial nerve**
- **Function**: (1) elbow flexion; (2) articularis cubitus fibers may assist in retracting anterior capsule during elbow flexion

MEDIAL ELBOW

Pronator Teres

- **Origin**: (1) humeral head: anterior + superior medial epicondyle; (2) ulnar head: coronoid process
- **Insertion**: broad insertion into lateral margin of radius at proximal–middle 1/3 junction, deep to brachioradialis
- **Innervation**: median nerve
- **Function**: forearm pronation

Flexor Carpi Radialis

- **Origin**: anterior and inferior aspect of medial epicondyle; immediately inferior to origin of pronator teres and common flexors
- **Insertion**: volar base of the index metacarpal +/− long finger metacarpal
- **Innervation**: median nerve
- **Function**: wrist flexion

Palmaris Longus

- **Origin**: medial epicondyle
- **Insertion**: palmar fascia/aponeurosis
- **Innervation**: median nerve
- **Function**: wrist flexion
- **Variable presence**: may be absent in ~15% (unilateral) and 7% (bilateral)
- Often, a source of tendon graft for reconstructive surgery

Flexor Digitorum Superficialis

- **Origin**: (1) medial epicondyle; (2) proximal/anterior 2/3 radius
- **Insertion**: palmar base of middle phalanx
- **Innervation**: median nerve
- **Function**: flexion of proximal interphalangeal joints of fingers; secondary wrist flexor

Flexor Carpi Ulnaris

- **Origin**: (1) posterior aspect of medial epicondyle; (2) proximal and medial ulna and medial coronoid
- **Insertion**: pisiform + pisohamate ligament + pisometacarpal ligament
- **Innervation**: ulnar nerve
- **Function**: wrist flexion and ulnar deviation; weak elbow flexion

LATERAL ELBOW

Brachioradialis

- **Origin**: lateral supracondylar margin of the distal 1/3 humerus
- **Insertion**: base of radial styloid
- **Innervation**: radial nerve
- **Function**: elbow flexion with forearm in neutral rotation
- Forms lateral contour of the cubital fossa
- Part of the "mobile wad of three" (BR, ECRL, ECRB)

Extensor Carpi Radialis Longus

- **Origin**: lateral supracondylar margin, distal to brachioradialis origin and immediately proximal to the common extensor origin
- **Insertion**: dorsal base of index finger metacarpal
- **Innervation**: radial nerve
- **Function**: (1) wrist extension/radial deviation; (2) elbow flexion
- Part of the "mobile wad of three" (BR, ECRL, ECRB)

Extensor Carpi Radialis Brevis

- **Origin**: lateral and superior aspect of lateral epicondyle, deep to ECRL and lateral to the common extensor origin
- Origin of ECRB is difficult to distinguish histologically from the EDC origin
- **Insertion**: dorsal base of long finger metacarpal
- **Innervation**: radial nerve or SBRN or PIN
- **Function**: (1) wrist extension; (2) elbow flexion
- Part of the "mobile wad of three" (BR, ECRL, ECRB)

Extensor Digitorum Communis

- **Origin**: anterior aspect of lateral epicondyle
- Origin of EDC is difficult to distinguish histologically from the ECRB origin
- **Insertion**: extensor apparatus of fingers
- **Innervation**: posterior interosseous nerve
- **Function**: (1) finger extension and abduction; (2) elbow flexion, particularly with forearm in pronation

Extensor Carpi Ulnaris

- **Origin**: humeral head (medial aspect of common extensor origin) and ulnar head (anconeus aponeurosis)
- **Insertion**: dorsal ulnar base of small finger metacarpal
- **Innervation**: posterior interosseous nerve
- **Function**: wrist extension/ulnar deviation

Supinator

- **Origin**: (1) lateral–anterior aspect of lateral epicondyle; (2) lateral collateral ligament; (3) crista supinatoris of proximal ulna
- **Insertion**: wraps as a broad insertion into anterior radius from slightly proximal to radial tuberosity to distal to the pronator teres insertion
- **Innervation**: radial nerve or posterior interosseous nerve
- **Function**: forearm supination

POSTERIOR ELBOW

Triceps Brachii

- **Origin**: (1) long head: infraglenoid tuberosity of the scapula; (2) lateral head: proximal lateral intramuscular septum/posterior humerus; (3) medial head: distal ½ posteromedial humerus
- **Insertion**: olecranon tip
- **Innervation**: radial nerve
- **Function**: elbow extension

Anconeus

- **Origin**: broad origin from posterior aspect of lateral epicondyle and lateral triceps fascia
- **Insertion**: lateral and dorsal aspect of proximal ulna, posterior to ECU
- **Innervation**: nerve to the Anconeus (terminating branch of radial nerve to medial head of triceps)
- **Function**: (1) elbow extension; (2) forearm supination; (3) elbow joint stabilizer

4.4   Arthroscopic Anatomy of the Elbow

PORTALS

- **Proximal anteromedial**
  - anterior to the intermuscular septum and 2 cm proximal to the medial epicondyle
  - *Primary neurovascular structure at risk:* ulnar nerve
- **Anteromedial**
  - 2 cm anterior and 2 cm distal to the medial epicondyle
  - *Primary neurovascular structure at risk:* medial antebrachial cutaneous nerve
- **Proximal anterolateral**
  - 1 to 2 cm proximal to the anterior epicondyle and directly on the anterior humerus
  - *Primary neurovascular structure at risk:* radial nerve
- **Direct lateral**
  - located at the "soft spot"; center of triangle formed by the lateral epicondyle + olecranon process + radial head
  - *Primary neurovascular structure at risk:* posterior antebrachial cutaneous nerve
- **Posterocentral**
  - midline; 3 cm proximal to olecranon tip
  - *Primary structures at risk:* posterior antebrachial cutaneous nerve + ulnar nerve
- **Posterolateral (Fig. 4.4-7)**
  - 2 to 3 cm proximal to olecranon tip at the lateral margin of the triceps
  - *Primary structure at risk:* medial and posterior antebrachial cutaneous nerves

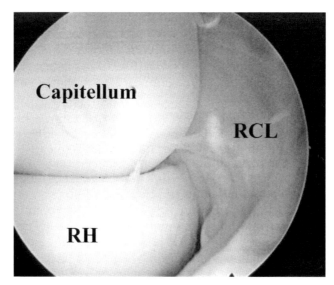

FIGURE 4.4-7 Arthroscopic anatomy: the capitellum *(Capitellum)* and radial head *(RH)* are identified. The lateral capsule and radial collateral ligament *(RCL)* are visualized.

RECOMMENDED READING

Atkinson WB, Elftman H. The carrying angle of the human arm as a secondary sex character. *Anat Rec.* 1945;91:49–52.

Beals RK. The normal carrying angle of the elbow. *Clin Orthop Relat Res.* 1976;119:194–196.

Caputo AE, Mazzocca AD, Santoro VM. The nonarticulating portion of the radial head: anatomic and clinical correlations for internal fixation. *J Hand Surg.* 1998;23A:1082–1090.

Eames MHA, Bain GI, Fogg QA, et al. Distal biceps tendon anatomy: a cadaveric study. *J Bone Joint Surg Am.* 2007;89A:1044–1049.

Field LD, Altchek DW, Warren RF, et al. Arthroscopic anatomy of the lateral elbow: a comparison of three portals. *Arthroscopy.* 1994;10:602–607.

Fuss FK. The ulnar collateral ligament of the human elbow joint. Anatomy, function and biomechanics. *J Anat.* 1991;175:203–212.

Johansson O. Capsular and ligament injuries of the elbow joint. A clinical and arthrographic study. *Acta Chir Scand Suppl.* 1962;287:1–159.

Lynch GJ, Meyers JF, Whipple TL, et al. Neurovascular anatomy and elbow arthroscopy: inherent risks. *Arthroscopy.* 1986;2:190–197.

Leonello DT, Galley IJ, Bain GI, et al. Brachialis muscle anatomy. A study in cadavers. *J Bone Joint Surg Am.* 2007;89:1293–1297.

Martin BF. The annular ligament of the superior radial ulnar joint. *J Anat.* 1958;52:473–482.

Martin BF. The oblique cord of the forearm. *J Anat.* 1958;52:609–615.

Miller CD, Jobe CM, Wright MH. Neuroanatomy in elbow arthroscopy. *J Shoulder Elbow Surg.* 1995;4:168–174.

Morrey BF. Anatomy of the Elbow Joint. In: Morrey BF, ed. *The Elbow and its Disorders.* 3rd ed. Philadelphia, PA: Saunders; 2000.

Morrey BF, An KN. Functional anatomy of the ligaments of the elbow. *Clin Orthop Relat Res.* 1985;201:84–90.

Morrey BF, Tanaka S, An KN. Valgus stability of the elbow. A definition of primary and secondary constraints. *Clin Orthop.* 1991;265:187–195.

O'Driscoll SW, Horii E, Morrey BF. Anatomy of the attachment of the medial ulnar collateral ligament. *J Hand Surg.* 1992;17:164–169.

O'Driscoll SW, Horii E, Morrey BF, et al. Anatomy of the ulnar part of the lateral collateral ligament of the elbow. *Clin Anat.* 1992;5:296–303.

O'Driscoll SW, Morrey BF, An KN. Intraarticular pressure and capacity of the elbow. *Arthroscopy.* 1990;6:100–103.

Ochi N, Ogura T, Hashizume H, et al. Anatomic relation between the medial collateral ligament of the elbow and the humero-ulnar joint axis. *J Shoulder Elbow Surg.* 1999;8:6–10.

Poehling GG, Whipple TL, Sisco L, et al. Elbow arthroscopy: a new technique. *Arthroscopy.* 1989;5:222–224.

Seki A, Olsen BS, Jensen SL, et al. Functional anatomy of the lateral collateral ligament complex of the elbow: configuration of Y and its role. *J Shoulder Elbow Surg.* 2002;11:53–59.

Spinner M, Kaplan EB. The quadrate ligament of the elbow: its relationship to the stability of the proximal radio-ulnar joint. *Acta Orthop Scand.* 1970;41:632–647.

Weiss AP, Hastings H II. The anatomy of the proximal radioulnar joint. *J Shoulder Elbow Surg.* 1992;1:193–199.

5 Neuroanatomy

5.1 Peripheral Nerve Anatomy—General

NEURAL ELEMENTS

- **Neuron**: contains a cell body that gives rise to dendrites and axons
- **Dendrites**: thin nerve processes that receive information from other nerve cells
- **Axons**: peripheral processes of the nerve cell body in the anterior horn (motor neuron) or in the dorsal root ganglion (sensory neuron); primary route of conduction from cell body via action potentials
- **Myelin**: fatty insulating sheath formed by the Schwann cells (glial cell type), which speeds conduction velocity of action potential
- **Schwann cells**: glial cell of the peripheral nervous system
- **Myelinated fibers**: axons are surrounded by Schwann cells and a myelin sheath
- **Nonmyelinated fibers**: large number of axons contained within the cytoplasm of a surrounding Schwann cell. Conduction is relatively slower.
- **Node of Ranvier**: gaps between Schwann cell segments of the myelin sheath which allow for efficient propagation of the action potential (Saltatory conduction)
- **Nerve fiber**: collection of axons and their Schwann cell sheaths; may be classified into three types (A, B, and C), based on fiber size and conduction velocity
- **Nerve fascicles/funiculus/fasciculi**
  - Smallest unit of the nerve that can be surgically manipulated, consisting of bundles or groups of fibers surrounded by perineurium
  - Collectively, form plexuses that are not simply parallel

NONNEURAL CONNECTIVE TISSUE

Endoneurium

- Loose collagenous matrix forming a bilaminar sheath surrounding the axon, Schwann cell, and myelin
- Composed of a collagenous matrix, including fibroblasts, mast cells, and capillaries

Perineurium

- Dense connective tissue sheath surrounding each fascicle
- High tensile strength
- Layers of flattened mesothelial cells presenting basement membranes on both sides act as a bidirectional diffusion barrier and are a blood–nerve barrier (extension of blood–brain barrier).
- Limits diffusion of epineural edema, such as occurs following injury

Epineurium

- Supportive connective tissue sheath containing multiple groups of fascicles
- **External epineurium** is the outer layer of the peripheral nerve.
- **Internal epineurium** surrounds individual fascicles.

VASCULAR SUPPLY

- Extensive intraneural vascular system, with vascular plexuses in all layers of the nerve, reinforced by segmental, regional extrinsic vessels

AXONAL TRANSPORT

- The neuron is a polarized cell with several intracellular transport systems.
- Molecular transport is dependent on adenosine triphosphate.
- **Anterograde transport**, from cell body to the terminus, is dependent on the carrier protein **kinesin**. There are slow (0.1 to 30 mm/day) and fast (up to 410 mm/day) anterograde transport mechanisms.
- **Retrograde transport**: permits protein recycling; it occurs at about one third the rate of anterograde transport and is dependent on the carrier protein **dynein**.
- **Myelin**: consists of 70% lipid and 30% protein
- **Resting membrane potential**: an electrical difference across the plasma membrane; the interior of the cell has a resting potential which is negative relative to the outside of the cell and is maintained by the Na^+/K^+ pump at between 50 and 80 mV.
- **Action potential**: permits the rapid transmission of electrical impulse over a long distance. Depolarization occurs when the graded potentials summate greater than the threshold.

5.2   Brachial Plexus (Fig. 5.2-1)

- Spinal nerve roots exit their respective intervertebral foramen and course between the intertransversalis muscles, posterior to the vertebral artery. They immediately divide into anterior primary rami (ventral rami) and posterior primary rami (dorsal rami).
- C5, C6, and C7 spinal nerves exit from above the C5, C6, and C7 vertebral bodies, respectively; C8 and T1 spinal nerves emerge from below the C7 and T1 vertebral bodies, respectively.
- **Dorsal rami** are **not** a part of the brachial plexus; they supply motor function and sensation to the posterior neck.
- **Ventral rami** are the spinal nerves that contribute to the brachial plexus.
  - The ventral rami exit the perivertebral column **between anterior and middle scalene muscles**.
- There is a low incidence of anomalies described for the brachial plexus (1% to 6%), although there is asymmetry in up to 38%.
- Brachial plexus typically includes contributions from C5 to T1.
  - **Prefixed plexus** includes C4 (approximately 20% of patients).
  - **Postfixed plexus** includes T2.
- The brachial plexus provides primary innervations to all muscles acting on the upper extremity, **except for the levator scapulae muscle** (primary from C3+C4, occasionally from dorsal scapular nerve) **and the trapezius muscle** (spinal accessory nerve—CN XI—and C3 + C4).

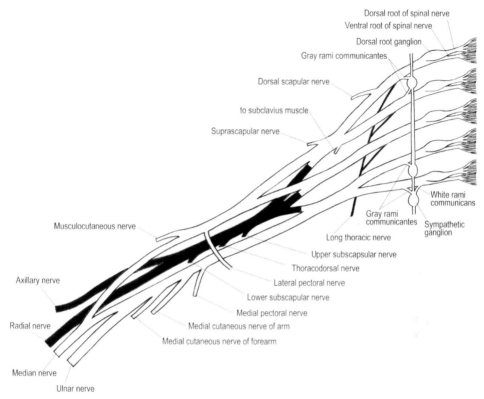

FIGURE 5.2-1 Illustration of the brachial plexus (right).

- The brachial plexus contains approximately **100,000 to 160,000 nerve fibers**.
- **Sympathetic contributions** to the brachial plexus include:
  - Gray rami communicate to spinal nerve roots.
  - Middle cervical ganglion to C5 and C6
  - Cervicothoracic ganglia to C7, C8, and T1
- **Horner syndrome** results from disruption of the C8 and T1 fibers that accompany the trigeminal nerve to the orbit, such as with C8 and T1 root avulsion injury. The loss of these contributions to the ciliary nerves result in a loss of function to the tarsal muscles, the orbital muscles of Müller, and the dilator muscles of the pupil. This results in the characteristic physical findings of Horner syndrome: **ptosis** (tarsal muscles), **enophthalmos** (Müller muscles), and **miosis** (dilator muscles of the pupil). Often, there is concomitant ipsilateral facial **anhydrosis**.
- **Roots** descend over the first rib toward the upper limb, posterior to the clavicle. The exception is T1 that must ascend over the first rib.
- The **posterior cervical triangle** is bordered by the trapezius muscle (posterior) + sternocleidomastoid muscle (anterior) + clavicle (inferior).
- Structures overlying the posterior cervical triangle include skin, platysma muscle, and deep fascia. The superclavicular nerves, nerve to the subclavius muscle, and the omohyoid muscle all cross superficially within the posterior cervical triangle.
- The **upper trunk** (C5 + C6), **middle trunk** (C7), and **lower trunk** (C8 + T1) are formed in the lower region of the posterior cervical triangle.
- **Erb's point**: where C5 and C6 unite at the anterolateral surface of the scalenus medius muscle.
- C8 and T1 unite at the inner border of the first rib, posterior to the scalenus anterior muscle and **Sibson fascia** (extension of the endothoracic fascia, or suprapleural

membrane, which attaches to the internal border of the first rib and transverse process of C7).

- The superficial cervical artery, a branch of the thyrocervical trunk, and the transverse cervical artery all cross the upper and middle trunks.
- Each of the trunks divide into **anterior and posterior divisions**.
- Anterior nerve fibers are oriented to supply the anterior/flexor limb; posterior fibers supply the posterior/extensor limb.
- The divisions are crossed by the **suprascapular artery**, a second branch of the thyrocervical trunk.
- Distal to the clavicle and posterior to the pectoralis minor, at the level of the uppermost portion of the serratus anterior muscle, the divisions contribute to the formation of the cords. **The cords are named based on their anatomic relationship to the axillary artery**:
  - Anterior divisions of upper and middle trunks → **lateral cord**
  - Anterior division of lower trunk → **medial cord**
  - Posterior division of upper, middle, and lower trunks → **posterior cord**
- At the posterior aspect of the pectoralis minor tendon, the cords of the brachial plexus are enveloped by the axillary sheath.
- The cords end in terminal branches:
  - Lateral cord → **musculocutaneous nerve + lateral root of the median nerve**
  - Medial cord → **ulnar nerve + medial root of the median nerve**
  - Posterior cord → **axillary nerve + radial nerve**
- Branches of the brachial plexus

Roots

- Branches arising from roots
  - **Dorsal scapular nerve**
    - Typically **C5**
    - Innervates the **rhomboid muscles**
    - Contributes to innervation of the levator scapulae
    - Travels on deep surface of levator scapulae to medial border of the scapula
  - **Long thoracic nerve**
    - Arises from the posterior aspect of **C5, C6, and C7** immediately distal to the intervertebral foramen
    - Contribution from C7 is often absent; branches from C5 and C6 join after piercing the scalenus medius muscle and C7 contributes more distally.
    - Runs posterior to the brachial plexus and axillary artery into the axilla, and is joined by the lateral thoracic artery at the superior margin of the serratus anterior muscle
    - Divides into branches to innervate the **serratus anterior muscle**
  - **Phrenic nerve**
    - **C3, C4, and C5**—primary contribution from C4
    - Runs from lateral to medial on the anterior surface of the anterior scalene muscle
    - May be followed proximally to identify the interval between the scalenus anterior and the scalenus medius muscles
    - **Innervates the diaphragm** after entering the thorax between the subclavian artery and vein
    - A root to the phrenic nerve may arise from the upper trunk and is known as the *accessory phrenic nerve.*

Trunks

- Branches arising from trunks

- **Nerve to subclavius muscle**
  - Arises from **anterior surface of the upper trunk**
  - Contains fibers from C4 and C5, occasionally C6
  - May arise independently (65%), or with a root to the phrenic nerve (29%), dorsal scapular (4%), or lateral pectoral nerve (2%)
  - Passes superficially to the subclavian vein to innervate the **subclavius muscle**
- **Suprascapular nerve**
  - Arises from **posterolateral upper trunk (C5, C6)** at Erb's point; may originate from the anterior or posterior division of the upper trunk. Occasional contribution from C4
  - Courses laterally in the interval between the omohyoid and trapezius muscles
  - Passes through the suprascapular notch, **inferior to the superior transverse scapular ligament**, to enter the supraspinous fossa. The nerve often divides into two branches before entering the supraspinatus and infraspinatus muscles.
  - From the supraspinous fossa it **innervates the supraspinatus muscle, the glenohumeral and acromioclavicular joints**.
  - Courses around the lateral border of the scapular spine with the suprascapular artery and descends **inferior to the inferior transverse scapular ligament** into the infraspinous fossa where it terminates, sending branches to the **infraspinatus muscle**

Divisions

- No branches exit plexus at this level.
- Each trunk contributes to both anterior and posterior divisions.

Cords

- Branches arising from cords
  Lateral Cord   (C4), C5 to C7
- **Lateral pectoral nerve**
  - May arise from a single root (23%) or from two to four roots (77%)
  - Contains fibers from C4 or C5 to C7
  - Arises laterally at the first part of the axillary artery, crosses anterior to the artery, and sends a branch to the medial pectoral nerve before piercing the clavipectoral fascia and dividing on the deep surface of the **pectoralis major muscle**.
- **Lateral root of the median nerve**
  - **A terminal branch of the lateral cord**; divides from the musculocutaneous nerve branch at the lateral border of the pectoralis minor muscle
  - Fibers (C5 to C7) will join with the medial root of the median nerve anterior (87%) or, occasionally posterior (13%), to the third part of the axillary artery.
- **Musculocutaneous nerve**
  - A terminal branch of the lateral cord
  - Contains fibers from C4 or C5 to C7; contributions from C8 and T1 in 7% only
  - Arises between the axillary artery and the coracobrachialis muscle
  - Pierces/innervates the **coracobrachialis muscle** and then descends between within the **biceps–brachialis** muscular interval, innervating both muscles
  - Provides articular branches to the elbow joint, then continues as the **lateral antebrachial cutaneous nerve** (provides sensation to anterolateral forearm) after piercing the lateral brachial fascia

- The **lateral antebrachial cutaneous** nerve emerges from the lateral aspect of the biceps tendon at the level of the intercondylar line.
- Occasionally, the lateral cord provides a **contribution to the ulnar nerve** (43%).

Medial Cord   (C7), C8 and T1, (T2)
- **Medial pectoral nerve**
  - A branch of the medial cord in 70%; 30% from the lower trunk
  - Usually contains fibers from C8 ± T1, and rarely C7
  - Arises posterior to axillary artery, then courses between artery and vein before communicating with the lateral pectoral nerve
  - Enters and innervates posterior surface of **pectoralis minor muscle**
  - Branches innervate **pectoralis major muscle**.
- **Medial brachial cutaneous nerve**
  - Smallest branch of the brachial plexus; contains fibers from T1 ± C8.
  - One or two branches; may communicate with intercostobrachial nerve
  - Arises from medial cord at lower border of pectoralis minor muscle and descends along the medial aspect of the brachial artery and basilica vein.
  - Pierces brachial fascia at the mid arm to supply **sensation to the medial brachium**
- **Medial antebrachial cutaneous nerve (MABCN)** (88% medial cord)
  - Arises from medial cord (80%) or lower trunk; contains fibers from T1 ± C8
  - May originate from above or below the medial brachial cutaneous nerve
  - Communicates with medial brachial nerve (4%) and ulnar nerve (6%)
  - Descends anteromedial to the brachial artery; pierces brachial fascia at mid arm with the basilic vein before dividing into anterior and posterior branches approximately 14.5 cm proximal to medial epicondyle (ME).
  - **The anterior branch** passes over ME or 2 to 3 cm anterior to ME and runs through the distal arm with the **basilic vein, passing anterior to the elbow between the biceps tendon and the medial humeral condyle**. It continues superficial to the FCU to the level of the wrist.
  - **The posterior branch** divides into one to four branches from 6 cm proximal to 4 cm distal to ME. Several articular branches to the elbow arise from the posterior branch.
  - The MABCN **provides sensation to the skin of the anterior brachium and the anteromedial antebrachium**.
- **Medial root of median nerve**
  - Terminal branch of the medial cord, containing fibers from C8 and T1; joins with lateral root of the median nerve anterior to the axillary artery
- **Ulnar nerve**
  - Major terminal branch of the medial cord; contains fibers from C7 or C8 to T1. May receive contributions from C5, C6, or T2 (33%)
  - Arises between axillary artery and vein and courses anterior to the teres major and latissimus muscles
  - Descends in arm **medial to the brachial artery**

Posterior Cord   C5 to C8, (T1)
- May be absent in up to 21%; radial and axillary nerves form independently from the posterior division when posterior cord is absent.
  - **Upper subscapular nerve**
    - Contains fibers from C5 ± C6
    - Courses posterior to axillary artery and pierces subscapular fascia to innervate the **subscapularis muscle**
  - **Lower subscapular nerve**
    - Contains fibers from C5 ± C6

- Occasionally arises from the axillary nerve
- Descends posterior to the axillary vein and subscapular vessels before dividing into two branches at the inferior margin of the subscapularis muscle. The branches innervate the **subscapularis muscle and the teres major muscle**.
- **Thoracodorsal nerve**
  - Originates between the upper and lower subscapular nerves
  - May arise from the radial, axillary, or subscapular nerves
  - Contains fibers from C7 only (50%), as well as from C5, C6, and C8 (50%)
  - Courses posterior to the axillary artery and descends with the **subscapular artery** in the posterior axilla
  - The subscapular artery divides into the thoracodorsal and circumflex scapular arteries; the thoracodorsal nerve follows its named artery and pierces and innervates the **latissimus dorsi muscle** 8 to 12 cm proximal to its insertion and 2 cm from its anterior border.
- **Axillary nerve**
  - Arises from posterior cord in 80%; may arise from posterior division of upper or upper and middle trunks
  - Contains fibers from C5 ± C6, rarely from C7
  - Arises at inferior margin of the subscapularis muscle; it sends an articular branch to the shoulder and joins the posterior humeral circumflex vessels and passes from anterior to posterior through the **quadrilateral space** before dividing into anterior and posterior branches.
  - The quadrilateral space is bordered by the following:
    - Superior: subscapularis muscle
    - Inferior: teres major muscle
    - Medial: long head of the triceps brachii muscle
    - Lateral: medial cortex of the proximal humeral diaphysis
  - In the axilla, the axillary nerve consists typically of one large fascicle; however, **as the nerve enters the quadrilateral space, three distinct group fascicular bundles are identified: (1) deltoid, (2) teres minor, and (3) superior lateral brachial cutaneous nerve.**
  - **Anterior branch**: courses with posterior humeral circumflex vessels around surgical neck of the humerus, sending motor branches to the anterior deltoid muscle, before dividing into cutaneous branches at the anterior margin of the deltoid muscle
  - **Posterior branch**: innervates the teres minor muscle and posterior deltoid
  - Posterior branch terminates as **superior lateral brachial cutaneous nerve.**
- **Radial nerve** (Fig. 5.2-2)
  - **Largest terminal branch of the brachial plexus**
  - From posterior cord (80%), or from the posterior divisions of the upper, upper and middle, or all three trunks
  - Contains fibers from C5 to C8, occasionally from T1
  - Branches from posterior cord posterior to the pectoralis minor muscle and descends posterior to the axillary artery, crossing anterior to the subscapularis, teres major, and latissimus dorsi muscles
  - Courses with the **profunda brachii artery** into the posterior compartment of the arm via the **triangular interval**
  - Borders of the triangular interval
    Superior: teres major
    Medial: long head of triceps brachii
    Lateral: humerus/lateral head of triceps

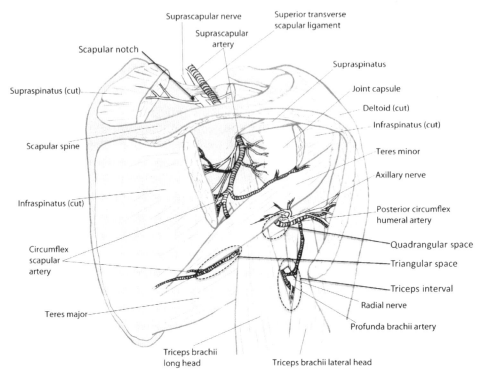

FIGURE 5.2-2 Illustration of the posterior aspect of the right shoulder, demonstrating the quadrangular space and the triangular space.

- The radial nerve/profunda brachii artery runs superior-medial to inferior-lateral in the brachium between the long and medial heads of the triceps muscle.
- The **posterior brachial cutaneous nerve**, which provides sensation to the posterior brachium, branches from the radial nerve in the axilla.

Branches

- **Axillary nerve**: formed from posterior cord
- **Musculocutaneous nerve**: formed from lateral cord
- **Radial nerve**: formed from posterior cord
- **Ulnar nerve**: formed from medial cord
- **Median nerve**: formed from medial and lateral cord

■ *Clinical Correlate:* The brachial plexus may be divided into supra- and infraclavicular portions. This distinction affects the surgical approach to the brachial plexus based on the need for osteotomy of the clavicle.

5.3   Radial Nerve (Figs. 5.3-1 to 5.3-5)

- Arises from the **posterior cord** of the brachial plexus (80%) (**C5 to C8; ±T1 [8%]**) or from the posterior divisions of the upper, upper and middle, or all three trunks
- Enters the brachium **anterior** to the subscapularis and triceps (long head) muscles, teres major, and latissimus dorsi tendons via the triangular interval
- Approximately 7 cm distal to the tip of the acromion, a branch of the radial nerve originates to supply the **long head of the triceps muscle**.

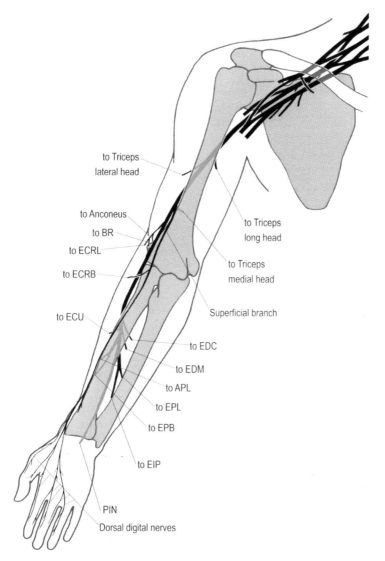

to Triceps
lateral head

to Anconeus

to BR

to ECRL

to ECRB

to ECU

to Triceps
long head

to Triceps
medial head

Superficial branch

to EDC

to EDM

to APL

to EPL

to EPB

to EIP

PIN

Dorsal digital nerves

FIGURE 5.3-1 Illustration of the anatomic course and branches of the radial nerve in the right upper extremity.

- Approximately 9 cm distal to the tip of the acromion is the origin of the branch to the medial portion of the **medial head of the triceps muscle**. This branch is known as the *ulnar collateral nerve* as it runs adjacent to the ulnar nerve itself while giving off multiple branches to the medial head of the triceps muscle.
- In the midbrachium, the radial nerve courses laterally with the **profunda brachii artery** between the medial and long heads of the triceps muscle and passes across the posterior humerus between the medial and lateral heads of the triceps muscle.
- Laterally, the nerve runs adjacent to, but not within, the spiral groove of the humerus, separated from the humerus by the medial head of the triceps. The posterior muscular branch of the radial nerve originates at the level of the spiral groove and provides motor innervations to the **medial and lateral heads of the triceps muscle and the anconeus muscle**.

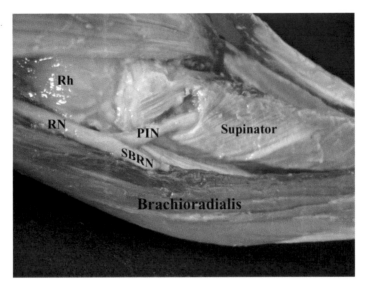

FIGURE 5.3-2 Division of the radial nerve *(RN)* in the proximity of the radiocapitellar joint and radial head *(Rh)*. The radial nerve divides into the posterior interosseous nerve *(PIN)* and the superficial branch of the radial nerve *(SBRN)*. The PIN enters the substance of the supinator muscle and runs distally, almost perpendicular to the fibers of the supinator muscle to innervate the extensor musculature of the forearm and to terminate as afferent fibers to supply the dorsal wrist capsule. The SBRN courses distally beneath the brachioradialis muscle, becoming superficial to the antebrachial fascia between the BR and ECRL tendons to provide sensory innervation to the dorsal and radial hand.

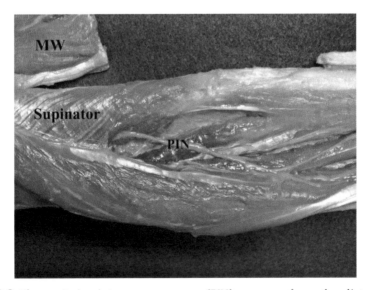

FIGURE 5.3-3 The posterior interosseous nerve *(PIN)* emerges from the distal edge of the supinator (superficial and deep heads), coursing distally to innervate, in order, the ECU-EDC-EDM-APL-EPL-EPB-EIP muscles. Here, the mobile wad *(MW)* of three—brachioradialis, extensor carpi radialis longus, and brevis—have been cut away. The supinator is seen to insert obliquely into the radius (at top).

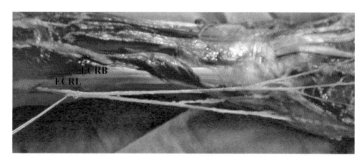

FIGURE 5.3-4 The superficial branch of the radial nerve *(SBRN)* is shown here, retracted from the forearm by a nerve hook, as it emerges from the brachioradialis and *ECRL* interval. The nerve pierces the forearm fascia approximately 9 cm from the radial styloid and divides into radial and ulnar divisions before arborizing over the dorsal and radial hand. *(ECRB,* extensor carpi radialis; *ECRL,* extensor carpi radialis longus).

- At the level of the deltoid tuberosity (insertion) of the humerus, the radial nerve lies directly posteriorly.
- The radial nerve pierces the lateral intermuscular septum with the radial collateral artery to enter the anterior compartment approximately **10 cm proximal to the lateral epicondyle**.
- One or more branches innervate the **lateral portion of the brachialis muscle**, and continue as articular branches of the elbow joint.
- In the distal brachium, the radial nerve courses **between the brachialis and the brachioradialis (BR) muscles** and **then between the brachialis and extensor carpi radialis (ECR) longus muscles**.

■ *Clinical Correlate:* The radial nerve may be compressed at one of four points in the brachium:
  - Fibrous band at the origin of the lateral head of the triceps
  - Lateral intermuscular septum in presence of a humerus fracture
  - Anomalous vascular structures or pathology in the axilla
  - Muscle anomaly: the accessory subscapularis-teres-latissimus muscle may compress the nerve at the subscapularis muscle.

- The nerve passes anterior to the lateral epicondyle, deep to the BR and ECR muscles and **divides into the superficial branch of the radial nerve (SBRN) and posterior interosseous nerve (PIN)**.
- The radial nerve bifurcates approximately 8.0 ± 1.9 cm distal to the lateral intermuscular septum, and 3.6 ± 0.7 cm proximal to the leading edge of the supinator muscle.
- The SBRN descends in the forearm deep to the BR muscle and radial to the radial artery. It pierces the deep fascia between the extensor carpi radialis longus (ECRL) and BR tendons approximately **9 cm** proximal to the radial styloid, courses superficial to the abductor pollicis longus (APL) and extensor pollicis brevis (EPB) tendons, and divides into radial and ulnar divisions before branching to provide sensation to the dorsal radial hand. An average of five to six branches may cross the wrist joint.
- The SBRN provides variable sensory innervation to the dorsal digits, as far distally as the base of the thumbnail, and to the PIP joint region of the fingers: 45% innervating the radial 2½ digits, 30% innervating the radial 3½ digits. The SBRN provides one to two branches to the lateral margin of the thenar eminence.

■ *Clinical Correlate:* **Cheiralgia paresthetica**, or **Wartenberg syndrome**, involves symptomatic compression of the SBRN between the fascia of the BR and ECRL (or split BR).

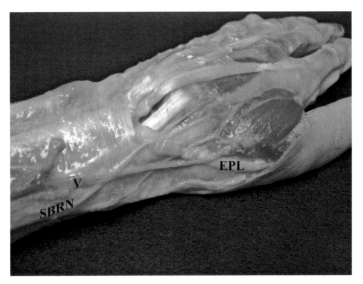

FIGURE 5.3-5 The superficial branch of the radial nerve *(SBRN)* divides into multiple branches at the radial wrist that are deep to the superficial venous structures *(V)*. This is in contradistinction to the distal branches of the lateral antebrachial cutaneous nerve which lie in the same plane as the superficial veins. Here, the SBRN branches are seen to pass directly over the dorsal surface of the extensor pollicis longus tendon *(EPL)*, placing these nerve branches at risk with dissection near to the EPL tendon.

- **The extensor carpi radialis bravis (ECRB) may be innervated by the radial nerve, the SBRN (45%), or the PIN**.
- The PIN courses perpendicularly through the deep and superficial heads of the supinator to lie between the APL/extensor carpi ulnaris (ECU) (deep) and extensor digiti minimi (EDM)/extensor digitorum communis (EDC) (superficially).
- The PIN crosses the radial shaft on average approximately 33 mm (forearm supinated) to 52 mm (forearm pronated) distal to the capitellum.
- The **Arcade of Frohse** is the fibrous, proximal leading edge of the supinator and may be a site of nerve compression.
- PIN arborizes into three short branches, each to ECU, EDM, and EDC, and into two longer branches to APL, extensor pollicis longus (EPL), EPB, and extensor indicis proprius (EIP).
- The classic order of innervation for PIN, distal to the leading edge of the supinator: **ECU-EDC-EDM-APL-EPL-EPB-EIP**
- The PIN innervates the extensor muscles of the forearm and courses distally deep to the fourth dorsal compartment with the posterior interosseous artery (PIA) **to terminate as afferent or sensory nerve branches supplying the dorsal wrist capsule**.

■ *Clinical Correlate:* The radial nerve may be compressed at one of five points in the radial tunnel:
  - The fascia adjacent to the radiocapitellar joint
  - The recurrent radial artery/Leash of Henry
  - The tendinous margin of the ECRB
  - The leading edge (fascial band present in 30%) of the supinator muscle (Arcade of Frohse). Typically found 5 cm distal to the lateral epicondyle.
  - The distal (dorsal) aspect of the supinator muscle

5.4 | Ulnar Nerve (Figs. 5.4-1 to 5.4-8)

- Arises from the **medial cord** of the brachial plexus. Consists of fibers from C7 or C8 to T1. May receive contributions from C5, C6, or T2 (33%).
- Descends posterior to the pectoralis major muscle and medial to the brachial artery.
- 8 cm proximal to the ME, the ulnar nerve and the **superior ulnar collateral artery** pierce the medial intermuscular septum and descend on the anterior surface of the medial head of the triceps muscle.
- The **Arcade of Struthers**, found in 20% to 70%, is a thick fascial band **formed by the medial intermuscular septum, internal brachial ligament, and triceps fascia** that spans from the medial head of the triceps muscle to the medial intermuscular septum and may be a site of nerve compression.
- The nerve passes from the posterior compartment of the brachium to the anterior compartment of the forearm via the **cubital tunnel**.

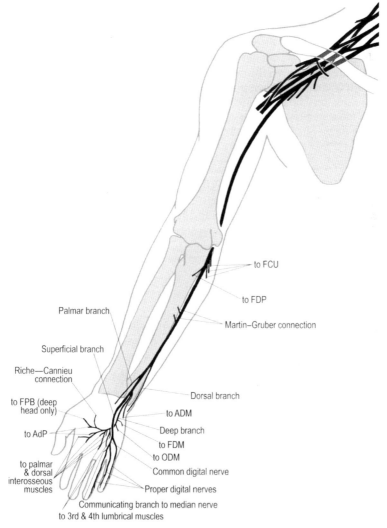

FIGURE 5.4-1 Illustration of the anatomic course and branches of the ulnar nerve in the right upper extremity.

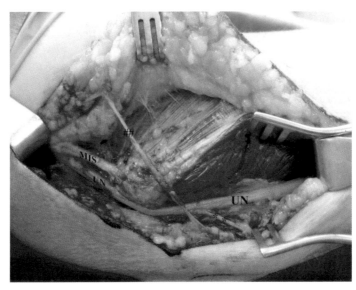

FIGURE 5.4-2 Intraoperative exposure of the ulnar nerve *(UN)* at the medial elbow after division of the overlying posterior brachial fascia and the fascial roof of the cubital tunnel (Osborne's fascia) and retraction of the heads of the flexor carpi ulnaris muscle distally. The ulnar nerve is located posterior to the medial intermuscular septum *(MIS)* and the medial epicondyle. Immediately anterior and superficial to the medial epicondyle, the medial antebrachial cutaneous nerve (MABCN) *(##)* courses from proximal to distal and is at risk for injury during local tissue dissection. The MABCN is a sensory nerve supplying the proximal posteromedial and medial forearm. Articular branches to the elbow may originate from the ulnar nerve within the cubital tunnel and the motor branches to the FCU muscle may vary in their number and origin (see text). A motor branch to the FCU is identified within the distal cubital tunnel *(**)*.

- The fibro-osseous cubital tunnel is bordered by the ulnar groove of the ME, a fascial arcade or arcuate ligament (spanning from the ME to the olecranon, connecting the humeral and ulnar heads of the FCU origin), and the FCU muscle bellies. The posterior and oblique bands of the ulnar collateral ligament comprise a portion of the cubital tunnel floor.

■ *Clinical Correlate:* An anomalous muscle, the **anconeus epitrochlearis**, may overlay the arcuate ligament.

- Articular branches to the elbow joint arise from within the cubital tunnel.
- Typically, the ulnar nerve innervates two forearm muscles: FCU and flexor digitorum profundus (FDP) (ring + small).
- Motor branches to FCU may arise 4 cm proximal to the elbow joint, from within the cubital tunnel, and from up to 10 cm distal to the ME. Most commonly, there are one to two motor branches to FCU; up to four branches have been reported. The proximal FCU branch may divide to innervate the FDP muscle.
- Typically, there is a single branch to FDP (80%) that arises approximately 3 cm distal to the ME and runs distally for about 2.5 cm before entering the muscle.
- The ulnar nerve runs between the FCU and flexor digitorum superficialis (FDS) in the forearm before emerging more superficially, radial to the FCU tendon.
- **The ulnar nerve is ulnar and volar to the ulnar artery.**
- The **dorsal sensory branch of the ulnar nerve (DSBUN)** branches approximately **6 cm** proximal to the ulnar head and courses distally and dorsally to supply the dorsal ulnar wrist and hand, the dorsal and proximal ring, and small fingers.

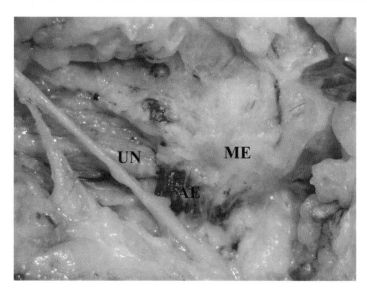

FIGURE 5.4-3 Intraoperative exposure of the ulnar nerve *(UN)* at the cubital tunnel region of the left elbow. The anomalous anconeus epitrochlearis muscle *(AE)* is identified superficial to the cubital tunnel, posterior to the medial epicondyle *(ME)*.

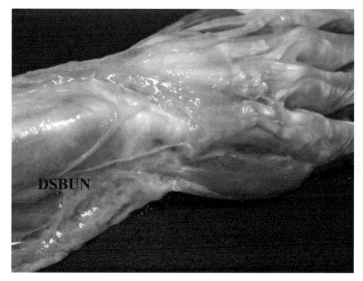

FIGURE 5.4-4 The dorsal sensory branch of the ulnar nerve *(DSBUN)* branches from the ulnar nerve approximately 6 cm proximal to the ulnar head and courses distally and dorsally to supply sensory innervation to the dorsal ulnar hand and the dorsal and proximal ring and small fingers. The nerve passes the ulnocarpal joint at approximately the level of the midsagittal aspect of the ulnar wrist. There is variability in the regions innervated by the superficial branch of the radial nerve and the DSBUN.

- At the wrist, the ulnar nerve is **45% motor/55% sensory**.
- For approximately **7.5 cm proximal to the level of the ulnar nerve bifurcation** into the superficial branch and the deep motor branch (which occurs in the distal ulnar tunnel, approximately 1 cm distal to the pisiform), the ulnar nerve may be identified as **two distinct groups of fascicles** traveling in a common epineural sheath. **The palmar radial fibers become the superficial branch and the dorsal ulnar fibers become the deep (motor) branch.**

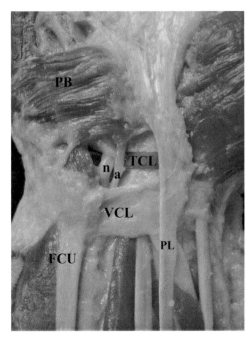

FIGURE 5.4-5 In the distal forearm, the ulnar artery and nerve descend in a fascial interval between the flexor carpi ulnaris *(FCU)* and the extrinsic digital flexors (FDS and FDP). The ulnar artery *(a)* remains dorsal and radial to the ulnar nerve *(n)* as it enters the distal ulnar tunnel at the leading edge of the volar carpal ligament *(VCL)*. The 4-cm long distal ulnar tunnel is divided into three zones (see text); the floor of zone 1 is the transverse carpal ligament *(TCL)*—the volar "roof" of the adjacent carpal tunnel. The palmaris brevis muscle *(PB)* is the transversely orientated muscle that serves as the roof of the distal ulnar tunnel in zone 2. Motor innervation of the PB is from two branches from the superficial or, otherwise, sensory branch of the ulnar nerve after its division in the distal ulnar tunnel. For reference, the palmaris longus *(PL)* is identified.

■ *Clinical Correlate:* The ulnar nerve may be compressed in the arm/at the elbow region at the following points:
- First rib
- Arcade of Struthers
  - A fibrous canal adjacent to the medial intermuscular septum from 4 to 10 cm proximal to the ME
  - Formed by the intramuscular septum, internal brachial ligament, and triceps fascia
- Medial head of the triceps. The internal brachial ligament, when present (~73%), supports the origin of the medial triceps.
- Anconeus epitrochlearis muscle
  - Present in 1% to 30% of limbs
  - Origin: ME
  - Insertion: medial border of olecranon
- Osborne's ligament (i.e., at the cubital tunnel proper)
- Ulnohumeral joint pathology (e.g., osteophytes, synovitis, and ganglion cyst)
- FCU muscle fascia and muscle belly

DISTAL ULNAR TUNNEL/GUYON'S CANAL—*THREE ZONES*

- The distal ulnar tunnel is approximately 4 to 4.5 cm in length.
- Entrance is at the proximal edge of the volar carpal ligament.

- Exit is at the distal margin of the fibrous arch of the hyopthenar muscles.
- Medial wall: FCU/pisiform/abductor digiti minimi (ADM)
- Lateral wall: transverse carpal ligament/hamate
- Roof: volar carpal ligament/palmaris brevis/hypothenar fat and fibrous tissue
- Floor: FDP tendons/transverse carpal ligament/pisohamate and pisotriquetral ligaments, opponens digiti minimi

Zone 1

- Begins at the proximal edge of volar carpal ligament (approximately 2 cm proximal to pisiform)
- Ends at nerve bifurcation, approximately 1 cm distal to pisiform
  - Palmar radial fibers become superficial branch.
  - Dorsal ulnar fibers become deep motor branch.
- Approximately 3 cm in length
- Roof: **volar carpal ligament**
- Floor: **transverse carpal ligament**
- Artery bifurcates distal to nerve

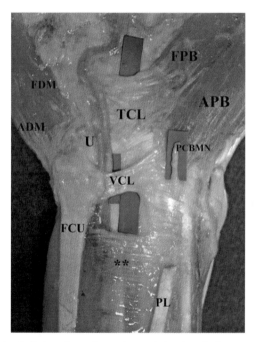

FIGURE 5.4-6 Landmarks defining the volar wrist and the distal ulnar tunnel and the carpal tunnel. The anterior compartment of the forearm is bound by the (volar) antebrachial fascia (**); the palmaris longus, cut away, is inconsistently present and is identified superficial to the deep fascia *(PL)* and the flexor carpi ulnaris *(FCU)* demarcates the ulnar margin of the distal forearm musculotendinous structures. The leading proximal edge of the volar carpal ligament *(VCL)* is the entrance to the distal ulnar tunnel or **Guyon's canal**. The ulnar nerve and artery *(U)* course distally and are volar to the transverse carpal ligament *(TCL)*. The abductor digiti minimi *(ADM)* originates from the pisiform and is dependent on its vascular supply from branches of the ulnar artery at its origin and should not be detached from the pisiform when considering an ADM transfer. The flexor digiti minimi *(FDM)* originates from the TCL and receives its innervation from the ulnar nerve in the distal Guyon's canal. Proximal to the TCL and the entrance to the carpal tunnel, the median nerve gives off its palmar cutaneous branch of the median nerve *(PCBMN)* which courses distally in its own tunnel/fascial compartment volar to the carpal tunnel to provide sensory innervation to the thenar eminence ± central palm. The PCBMN (cut) is seen here to course over the base of the thenar eminence and abductor pollicis brevis muscle *(APB)*. The flexor pollicis brevis muscle *(FPB)* is identified originating on the TCL and distal to the APB.

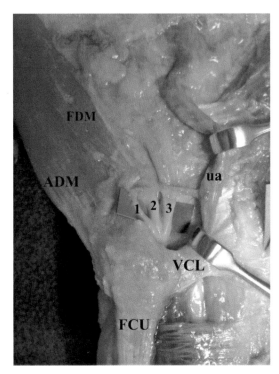

FIGURE 5.4-7 The distal ulnar tunnel has been exposed distal to the volar carpal ligament *(VCL)* and the ulnar artery *(ua)* has been retracted radially. In the midportion of the distal ulnar tunnel, the ulnar nerve divides into the superficial palmar cutaneous branch *(3)* and deep motor branch *(2)*. The superficial branch sends two motor branches to the palmaris brevis muscle and then remains sensory, innervating the ulnar border of the distal hand and dividing into the proper ulnar digital nerve to the small finger and the common digital nerve to the ring-small webspace. The deep motor branch sends a branch *(1)* to the abductor digiti minimi *(ADM)* and then courses around the hook of the hamate to innervate the flexor digiti minimi *(FDM)* and opponens digiti minimi, then courses across the palm with the ulnar artery (deep palmar arch) to innervate the interossei, third + fourth lumbricals, adductor pollicis, and flexor pollicis brevis. FCU, flexor carpi ulnaris.

Zone 2

- Roof: **palmaris brevis**
- Floor: **pisohamate + pisometacarpal ligaments**
- **Deep motor branch** passes around the hook of the hamate and between (and innervates) the ADM and flexor digiti minimi muscles, piercing the opponens digiti minimi to follow the deep palmar arch and to innervate (typically) the interossei muscles, third + fourth lumbricals, adductor pollicis, and flexor pollicis brevis (FPB) muscles.

Zone 3

- **Sensory branch**: remains superficial; **innervates palmaris brevis muscle** and is sensory to small finger and (typically) to ulnar ring finger

■ *Clinical Correlate:* The ulnar nerve may be compressed in the wrist/hand at the following points:
- Palmaris brevis muscle
- Fibrous origin of the flexor digiti minimi
- Ulnar artery aneurysm or thrombosis
- Distal ulnar tunnel ganglia

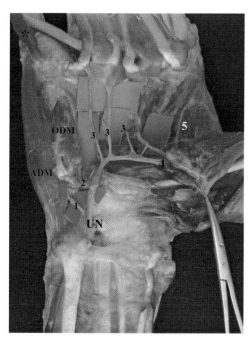

FIGURE 5.4-8 Course of the deep motor branch of the ulnar nerve *(UN)*. The extrinsic flexor tendons and lumbricals have been reflected distally. Motor innervation includes *(1)* abductor digiti minimi—*ADM*; *(*)* flexor digiti minimi—FDM, reflected distally; *(2)* opponens digiti minimi—*ODM*; *(3)* interossei muscles; *(4)* adductor pollicis muscle (reflected proximally) and flexor pollicis brevis muscle (not shown); *(5)* first dorsal interosseous muscle.

5.5   Median Nerve (Figs. 5.5-1 to 5.5-9)

- Arises from **medial + lateral cords** of the brachial plexus and contains fibers from **C5 to T1** (C5 contribution is inconsistent)
- Formed anterior or posterior to the third portion of the axillary artery
- Descends lateral to the brachial artery in brachialis/biceps interval.
- Located anteromedial to the brachialis muscle and posteromedial to the biceps brachii muscle until the level of the coracobrachialis insertion when the nerve crosses anterior to the brachial artery to become situated medial to the vessel.
- The **supracondylar process** (present in approximately 1%) is 3 to 5 cm proximal to the ME and projects anteromedially. The **Ligament of Struthers** joins the supracondylar process to the ME and forms a fibro-osseous tunnel through which the median nerve passes—the nerve is medial to the brachial artery at this level.
- Within the antecubital fossa, the median nerve lies anterior to the brachialis muscle and deep to the lacertus fibrosus, and remains **medial to the brachial artery**.
- It enters the forearm between the ulnar and humeral heads of the pronator teres.
- **It is separated from the deeper ulnar artery by the deep (humeral) head of the pronator teres in the proximal forearm.**
- In 82% the median nerve lies between the deep and superficial head of the pronator teres.
  - In ~9% the deep head of pronator teres is absent and the median nerve and ulnar artery travel deep to the superficial head.
  - In ~7% the median nerve travels deep to both heads of pronator teres.
  - In ~2% the median nerve travels through the substance of the superficial head of the pronator teres.

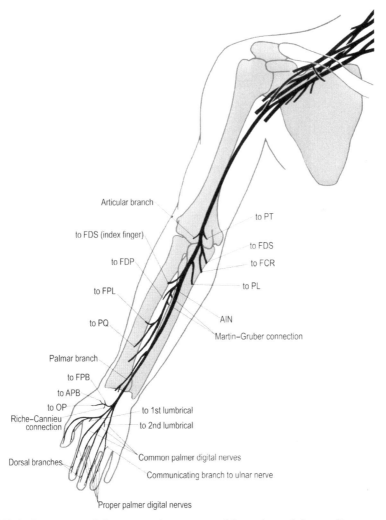

FIGURE 5.5-1 Illustration of the anatomic course and branches of the median nerve in the right upper extremity.

- The median nerve runs distally between the FDS and FDP muscles, typically in the FDS epimysium, although it may course within the FDS muscle substance.

■ *Clinical Correlate:* The median nerve may be compressed proximally with a resulting pain syndrome without objective motor or sensory findings: pronator syndrome.

Potential sites of nerve compression include:
- Pectoralis minor muscle
- Anomalous or pathologic axillary vascular structures
- Supracondylar process (3 cm proximal to ME)/Ligament of Struthers
- Gantzer's muscle: anomalous muscle arising from medial humeral condyle and inserting into flexor pollicis longus (FPL). It is dorsal to the anterior interosseous nerve (AIN). Present in 45% of limbs
- Lacertus fibrosis
- Humeral and ulnar heads of pronator teres
- FDS aponeurotic arch

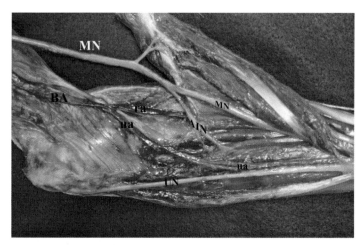

FIGURE 5.5-2 Volar and medial view of the elbow and proximal 2/3 forearm. The flexor digitorum superficialis (FDS) and pronator teres (PT) and median nerve *(MN)* have been elevated, exposing the brachial artery *(BA)* as it lies on the volar surface of the brachialis muscle and its division into the radial artery *(ra)* and ulnar artery *(ua)*. The ulnar artery courses distally and ulnarly toward the ulnar nerve *(UN)*; the artery remains radial to the nerve throughout the forearm and wrist. The median nerve innervates the FDS muscle (branch elevated with FDS muscle, in photo) and descends the forearm in the FDS/FDP muscular interval, often contained within the epimysium of the FDS, although has been described to run within the muscular substance of the FDS. The anterior interosseous nerve *(AIN)* branches just distal to the FDS muscular arch and typically innervates the FDP (index and long), the flexor pollicis longus (FPL), and pronator quadratus (PQ) muscles. A branch to the FDP from the AIN is seen here. The deep head of the pronator teres (when present), which has been elevated in this figure, separates the AIN from the ulnar artery.

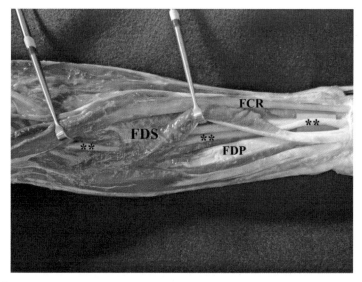

FIGURE 5.5-3 Volar forearm and course of the median nerve *(**)*. The median nerve courses between the humeral and ulnar heads of the pronator teres muscle before descending in the forearm between the flexor digitorum superficialis *(FDS)* and flexor digitorum profundus *(FDP)* muscles. The nerve may run within the substance of the FDS, but is most commonly within the dorsal epimysium of the FDS. The flexor carpi radialis *(FCR)* and FDS are both retracted to allow for visualization of the median nerve. Distally, the median nerve is identified in the FCR–FDS interval.

- Anomalous muscles in distal ⅓ forearm:
  - Palmaris profundus
        Origin: radius, proximal to FPL
        Insertion: transverse carpal ligament
  - Flexor carpi radialis (FCR) brevis
        Origin: near proximal origin of FPL
        Insertion: joins FCR
  - Ulnar collateral artery and aberrant branches of radial artery to AIN
  - Carpal tunnel
  - Palmar cutaneous branch within the transverse retinacular ligament
- The **AIN** typically branches immediately distal to the FDS arch and innervates the FDP (index and long fingers), FPL, and the pronator quadratus (PQ).
- The AIN courses distally on the interosseous membrane, often radial to the anterior interosseous artery (80%), and passes dorsal to the PQ muscle innervating the PQ via several motor branches. The terminal sensory portion of the AIN is distinguished only after the last motor branch, approximately 2 cm proximal to the ulnar head, and tunnels distally through a foramen in the distal and radial PQ. The AIN arborizes and terminates as afferent fibers supplying the periosteum of the volar lip of the distal radius and the volar wrist capsule, occasionally to the volar distal radioulnar joint capsule.

■ *Clinical Correlate:* **Anterior interosseous nerve syndrome** is a motor nerve compression syndrome with the primary clinical findings of absent/weak motor function of the FPL and FDP to the index finger.

- 5 cm proximal to the wrist crease, the median nerve runs more superficially in the FDS–FCR interval.
- The **palmar cutaneous branch of the median nerve (PCBMN)** arises approximately 5 to 7 cm proximal to the volar wrist crease and travels within the median nerve epineurium for approximately 16 to 25 mm. The PCBMN runs in the palmaris longus (PL)–FCR interval until it passes superficial to the transverse carpal ligament in

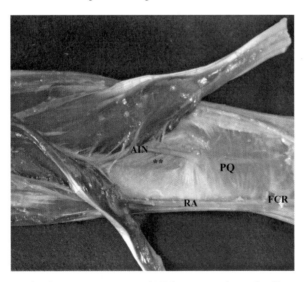

FIGURE 5.5-4 The anterior interosseous nerve *(AIN)* emerges from the flexor digitorum profundus (FDP) muscle and runs on the volar surface of the interosseous membrane *(**)* dorsal to the pronator quadratus *(PQ)* with the anterior interosseous artery. The AIN supplies motor innervation to the PQ muscle and terminates as afferent branches supplying the volar wrist capsule. Flexor carpi radialis distal tendon *(FCR)*; radial artery *(RA)*.

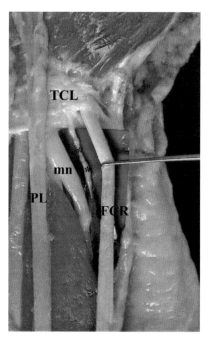

FIGURE 5.5-5 The palmar cutaneous branch of the median nerve (PCBMN) (******) arises approximately 5 to 7 cm proximal to the volar wrist crease and travels within the median nerve epineurium for approximately 2 cm. The PCBMN runs in the palmaris longus (**PL**)–**FCR** interval until it passes superficial to the transverse carpal ligament *(TCL)* in its own compartment to supply sensory innervation to the thenar eminence. Also, it sends superficial sensory branches to the skin overlying the carpal tunnel. **mn** = median nerve.

its own compartment to supply sensory innervation to the thenar eminence. Also, it sends superficial sensory branches to the skin overlying the carpal tunnel. The PCBMN comprises 2% of median nerve fibers.

■ *Clinical Correlate:* While the sensation provided by the PCBMN is not vital to hand function, injury to the nerve may result in causalgia with a painful neuroma.

- At the carpal tunnel, the median nerve is **94% sensory/6% motor**.
- **Distribution of motor fascicles** within the median nerve at the carpal tunnel:
  - 60% radial
  - 18% volar radial
  - 22% central
- **Traditional innervation pattern of the recurrent motor branch** (approximately 45% incidence) includes one main thenar trunk with three terminal branches, one each to the abductor pollicis brevis (APB), FPB, and opponens pollicis (OP).
- **Variations of recurrent motor branch innervation** have been described, however, including
  - 30% with two terminal branches to APB and FPB
  - 40% independent (main) branch to APB and OP
  - 75% had an **accessory thenar nerve** arising from either the first common digital nerve (25%) or the radial proper digital nerve to the thumb (50%).
- **Variations in the origin of the recurrent motor branch** have been described.
  - 46% extraligamentous
  - 31% subligamentous
  - 23% transligamentous

- Distal to the carpal tunnel, the median nerve branches into **radial and ulnar divisions**.
- The radial division branches into the common digital nerve to the thumb and the proper digital nerve to the radial index finger.
- The ulnar division divides into the common digital nerves to the second and third web spaces.
- Variations in the sensory innervation to the thumb and index finger
  - (69%) Radial digital nerve (RDN) to thumb + common digital nerve to first web space (which divides into ulnar digital nerve (UDN) to thumb and RDN to index finger).
  - (25%) Each branch is an independent branch from the median nerve (RDN to thumb + UDN to thumb + RDN to index).
  - (6%) Common digital nerve to thumb + RDN to index finger
- **The first and second lumbrical muscles are innervated by branches of the common digital nerves.**
- Common digital nerves are dorsal to the superficial palmar arch and palmar to the flexor tendons in the palm.
- The proper digital nerves become **palmar** to the digital arteries at the level of the metacarpal necks and continue this relationship into the fingers.

CARPAL TUNNEL

Floor: carpus/palmar radiocarpal ligaments
Roof: transverse carpal ligament
Radial border: scaphoid and trapezium
Ulnar border: triquetrum and hamate
Average volume: 5.84 mL; increases approximately 25% following CTR"

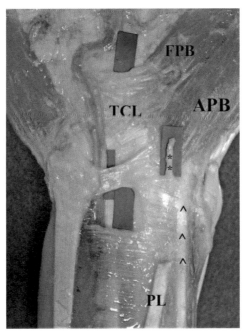

FIGURE 5.5-6 Proximal to the transverse carpal ligament *(TCL)* and the entrance to the carpal tunnel, the median nerve gives off its palmar cutaneous branch of the median nerve *(**)* which courses distally in its own tunnel/fascial compartment volar to the carpal tunnel to provide sensory innervation to the thenar eminence ± central palm. The PCBMN (cut) is seen here to course over the base of the thenar eminence and abductor pollicis brevis muscle *(APB)*. The flexor pollicis brevis muscle *(FPB)* is identified originating on the TCL and distal to the APB. PL = palmaris longus tendon; ^ = flexor carpi radialis (FCR), deep to the antebrachial fascia.

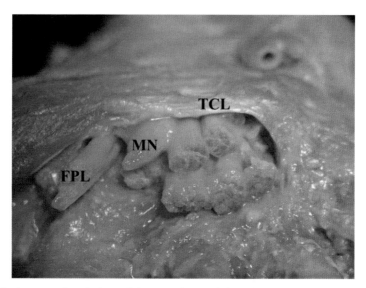

FIGURE 5.5-7 Cross-sectional view of the carpal tunnel demonstrating the relationship of the ulnar artery and nerve at the distal ulnar tunnel (background) to the transverse carpal ligament *(TCL)* and the contents of the carpal tunnel. Note that the ulnar nerve and artery are superficial to the TCL and are enclosed by the volar carpal ligament. The median nerve *(MN)* is most commonly found volar and radial relative to the contents of the carpal canal which include the flexor pollicis longus tendon *(FPL)* and the extrinsic finger flexor tendons (FDS and FDP). The recurrent motor branch of the median nerve is identified at the distal margin of the TCL, entering the abductor pollicis brevis muscle.

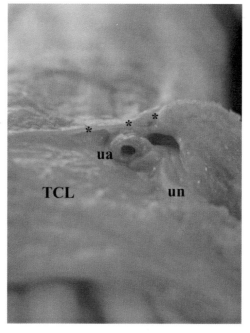

FIGURE 5.5-8 Close-up, oblique view of the distal ulnar artery and nerve to demonstrate the relationship of the distal ulnar tunnel and the carpal tunnel. The ulnar nerve *(un)* is dorsal and ulnar to the ulnar artery *(ua)*; both structures run superficial/volar to the transverse carpal ligament *(TCL)* and are dorsal to the volar carpal ligament (***).

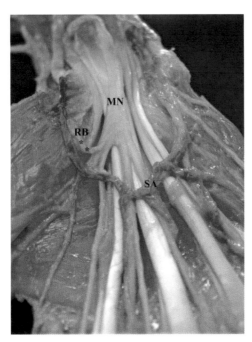

FIGURE 5.5-9 Oblique view of the carpal canal and proximal palm following removal of the transverse carpal ligament and fascial supporting structures. (Top = proximal) The median nerve *(MN)* is typically volar to the extrinsic digital flexor tendons and its relationship to the superficial palmar arterial arch *(SA)* is demonstrated. This "complete" SA, with its contributions from the palmar branch of the radial artery (seen here, coursing through the superficial muscle fibers of the thenar eminence) and the ulnar artery, is volar to the MN and the flexor tendons. The MN branches, including the recurrent motor branch *(RB**)*, are dorsal to the SA until the distal palm at which point the common digital nerves become volar/palmar to the digital arteries.

Transverse Carpal Ligament

- Spans from **pisiform and hook of hamate to scaphoid tubercle and trapezial ridge**
- Average dimensions: 22 mm wide, 26 mm long

■ *Clinical Correlate:* Carpal tunnel syndrome (CTS) is a compressive neuropathy of the median nerve within the carpal tunnel. Common symptoms include numbness and tingling, or paresthesias, pain, nocturnal awakening, and muscular weakness.

Motor branches of the median nerve (descending in forearm)	
Pronator teres →	arises 7 cm proximal to 2.3 cm distal to ME
	(one branch 30%, two branches 45%, and three branches 25%)
FCR →	proximal to AIN (one branch)
PL →	proximal to AIN (one branch)
FDS →	proximal to AIN (two to seven branches)
AIN →	5 cm distal to ME, often just distal to FDS arch
	Dorsoradial portion of median nerve
	Innervates FDP (index), FPL, PQ
Recurrent motor →	variable branching pattern (see above)

5.6   Nerve Anomalies

MARTIN–GRUBER CONNECTION

- Connection between the median and ulnar nerves in the proximal 1/3 forearm proximal to AIN branch, or distally within the FDP muscle (between ulnar nerve and AIN)
- Contains motor, sensory, or mixed fibers from median nerve or AIN
- Occurs in approximately 10% to 25%
  - Type I (60%): median motor branches to ulnar nerve and innervate muscles usually innervated by median nerve
  - Type II (35%): median motor branches to ulnar nerve and innervate muscles usually innervated by ulnar nerve
  - Type III (3%): ulnar motor branches to median nerve and innervate muscles usually innervated by median nerve
  - Type IV (2%): ulnar motor branches to median nerve and innervate muscles usually innervated by ulnar nerve

RICHE–CANNIEU CONNECTION

- Connection between the median and ulnar nerves within the substance of the FPB
- Median nerve may innervate third or all lumbricals
- Occurs in approximately 50% to 77%

RECOMMENDED READING

Abrams RA, Brown RA, Botte MJ. The superficial branch of the radial nerve: an anatomic study with surgical implications. *J Hand Surg.* 1992;17A:1037–1041.

Abrams RA, Ziets RJ, Lieber RL, et al. Anatomy of the radial nerve motor branches in the forearm. *J Hand Surg.* 1997;22A:232–237.

Auerbach DM, Collins ED, Kunkle KL, et al. The radial sensory nerve. *Clin Orthop Rel Res.* 1994; 308:241–249.

Bas H, Kleinert JM. Anatomic variations in sensory innervations of the hand and digits. *J Hand Surg.* 1999;24A:1171–1184.

Bourne MH, Wood MB, Carmichael SW. Locating the lateral antebrachial cutaneous nerve. *J Hand Surg.* 1987;12A:697–699.

Carlan D, Pratt J, Patterson JM, et al. The radial nerve in the brachium: an anatomic study in human cadavers. *J Hand Surg.* 2007;32A:1177–1182.

Diliberti T, Botte MJ, Abrams RA. Anatomical considerations regarding the posterior interosseous nerve during posterolateral approaches to the proximal part of the radius. *J Bone Joint Surg.* 2000;82A:809–813.

Eversmann WW. Proximal median nerve compression. *Hand Clin.* 1992;8:307–315.

Falconer D, Spinner M. Anatomic variations in the motor and sensory supply of the thumb. *Clin Orthop Relat Res.* 1985;(195):83–96.

Gelberman RH. *Operative Nerve Repair and Reconstruction.* Philadelphia, PA: JB Lippincott; 1991.

Gross MS, Gelberman RH. The anatomy of the distal ulnar tunnel. *Clin Orthop Relat Res.* 1985; (196):238–247.

Grafe MW, Kim PD, Rosenwasser MP, et al. Wrist denervation and the anterior interosseous nerve: anatomic considerations. *J Hand Surg.* 2005;30A:1221–1225.

Harris W. The true form of the brachial plexus and its motor distribution. *J Anat Physiol.* 1904;38:399–422.

Hollinshead WH. Anatomy for Surgeons. Vol. 3. *The Back and Limbs.* 3rd ed. New York, NY: Harper & Row; 1982.

Horwitz MT, Tocantins LM. An anatomic study of the role of the long thoracic nerve and the related scapular bursae in the pathogenesis of local paralysis of the serratus anterior muscle. *Anat Rec.* 1938;71:375–385.

Jamieson RW, Anson BJ. The relation of the median nerve to the heads of origin of the pronator teres muscle: a study of 300 specimens. *Q Bull Northwest Univ Med School.* 1952;26:34–35.

Jolley BJ, Stern PJ, Starling T. Patterns of median nerve sensory innervation to the thumb and index finger: an anatomic study. *J Hand Surg.* 1997;22A:228–231.

Kameda Y. An anomalous muscle (accessory subscapularis-teres-latissimus) in the axilla penetrating the brachial plexus in man. *Acta Anat (Basel).* 1976;96:513–533.

Kerr AT. The brachial plexus of nerves in man, the variations in its formation and its branches. *Am J Anat.* 1918;23:285–395.

Kimura I, Ayyar DR, Lippmann SM. Electrophysiological verification of the ulnar to median nerve communications in the hand and forearm. *Tohoku J Exp Med.* 1983;141:269–274.

Konig PS, Hage JJ, Bloem JJ, et al. Variations of the ulnar nerve and ulnar artery in Guyon's canal: a cadaveric study. *J Hand Surg.* 1994;19A:617–622.

Lanz U. Anatomical variations of the median nerve in the carpal tunnel. *J Hand Surg.* 1977;2A: 44–53.

Larkin FC. Accessory phrenic nerve. *J Anat Physiol.* 1889;23:340.

Laroy V, Spaans F, Reulen J. The sensory innervations pattern of the fingers. *J Neurol.* 1998;245: 294–298.

Linell EA. The distribution of nerves in the upper limb with reference to variabilities and their clinical significance. *J Anat.* 1921;55:79–112.

Leibovic SJ, Hastings H II. Martin-Gruber revisited. *J Hand Surg.* 1992;17A:47–53.

Lisanti M, Rosati M, Maltinti M. Ulnar nerve entrapment in Guyon's tunnel by an anomalous palmaris longus muscle with a persisting median artery. *Acta Orthop Belg.* 2001;67:399–402.

Lourie GM, King J, Kleinman WB. The transverse radioulnar branch from the dorsal sensory ulnar nerve: its clinical and anatomical significance further defined. *J Hand Surg.* 1994;19A: 241–245.

Lundborg G. The intrinsic vascularization of human peripheral nerves: structural and functional aspects. *J Hand Surg.* 1979;4:34–41.

Lundborg G, Dahlin LB. Anatomy, function, and pathophysiology of peripheral nerves and nerve compression. *Hand Clin.* 1996;12:185–193.

Mackinnon SE, Dellon AL. Anatomic investigations of nerves at the wrist: I. Orientation of the motor fascicle of the median nerve in the carpal tunnel. *Ann Plast Surg.* 1988;21:32–35.

Mackinnon SE, Dellon AL. The overlap pattern of the lateral antebrachial cutaneous nerve and the superficial branch of the radial nerve. *J Hand Surg Am.* 1985;10A:522–526.

Masear VR, Meyer RD, Pichora DR. Surgical anatomy of the medial antebrachial cutaneous nerve. *J Hand Surg.* 1989;14A:267–271.

Miller R. Observations upon the arrangement of the axillary artery and brachial plexus. *Amer J Anat.* 1939;64:143–163.

Olave E, Prates JC, Del Sol M, et al. Distribution patterns of the muscular branch of the median nerve in the thenar region. *J Anat.* 1995;186(pt 2):441–446.

Ozer Y, Grossman JA, Gilbert A. Anatomic observations on the suprascapular nerve. *Hand Clin.* 1995;11:539–544.

Sunderland S. The innervations of the flexor digitorum profundus and lumbrical muscles. *Anat Rec.* 1945;93:317–321.

Taleisnik J. The palmar cutaneous branch of the median nerve and the approach to the carpal tunnel. *J Bone Joint Surg.* 1973;55A:1212–1217.

Thomas SJ, Yakin DE, Parry BR, et al. The anatomical relationship between the posterior interosseous nerve and the supinator muscle. *J Hand Surg.* 2000;25A:936–941.

von Schroeder HP, Scheker LR. Redefining the "Arcade of Struthers." *J Hand Surg.* 2003;28A: 1018–1021.

Wehrli L, Oberlin C. The internal brachial ligament versus the arcade of Struthers: an anatomical study. *Plast Reconstr Surg.* 2005;115:471–477.

Whitson RO. Relation of the radial nerve to the shaft of the humerus. *J Bone Joint Surg.* 1954;36-A: 85–88.

6 Vascular Anatomy of the Upper Extremity

SUBCLAVIAN ARTERY

- Defined as artery **extending to the lateral margin of the first rib**
- Divided into three parts, based on relationship to anterior scalene muscle:
  - Part 1—*origin (innominate artery on right, from arch of aorta on left) to medial border of anterior scalene muscle*
    - Three branches:
      - **Vertebral artery**
      - **Internal mammary artery**
      - **Thyrocervical trunk**
        - Transverse cervical artery (TCA) (superior) and suprascapular artery (inferior) as independent branches (70%)
        - TCA and suprascapular artery arise as common branch (30%)
        - TCA divides into superficial branch to trapezius + deep TCA
        - Deep TCA is renamed as dorsal scapular artery if it arises from subclavian artery instead of TCA
  - Part 2—*lies directly posterior to the anterior scalene muscle*
    - One branch
      - **Costocervical trunk**
  - Part 3—*lateral border of anterior scalene muscle to lateral first rib*
    - One branch
      - **Dorsal scapular artery**
        - May arise from second part of subclavian artery or from TCA

AXILLARY ARTERY (Figs. 6-1 and 6-2)

- Defined as artery **extending from lateral margin of first rib to the inferior border of the teres major muscle**
- Divided into three parts, based on relationship to pectoralis minor muscle:
  - First part (one major branch)
    - Superior/medial to pectoralis minor muscle
    - Branches:
      1. **Supreme thoracic artery**—supplies intercostals spaces 1, 2 ± 3
  - Second part (two major branches)
    - Deep to the pectoralis minor muscle
    - Branches:
      1. **Thoracoacromial artery**—pierces clavipectoral fascia; four branches:
         1. Pectoral branch—courses between pectoralis major and minor muscles; supplies pectoralis major only in 86%
         2. Deltoid branch—perfuses head of pectoralis major and anterior deltoid muscles

  3. Acromial branch
  4. Clavicular branch

  2. Lateral thoracic artery
  - Most variable in its origin
  - 25% origin from subscapular artery; may arise from pectoral branch
  - Supplies pectoralis minor and serratus anterior muscles, intercostals spaces 3 to 5
- Third part (three major branches)
  - Lateral to the pectoralis minor muscle
  - Branches:
    1. Subscapular artery
    - Largest branch arising from axillary artery; courses caudally on anterior surface of subscapularis muscle
    - **Circumflex scapular artery** is first major branch; it runs through the triangular space

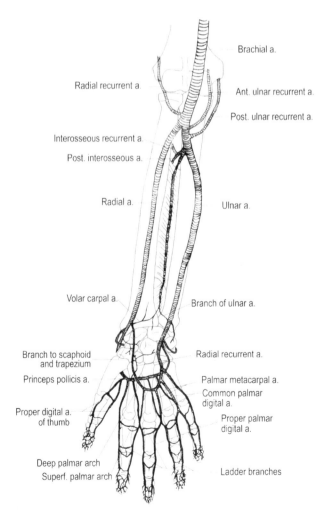

FIGURE 6.1 Illustration of the primary arterial anatomy of the volar forearm, wrist, and hand.

2. Anterior humeral circumflex artery
  - *Primary vascular supply to the humeral head*
  - Arises with, or slightly distal to posterior humeral circumflex artery, 1 cm distal to inferior border of pectoralis major muscle
  - Passes deep to biceps tendon and ascends to humeral head along lateral biceps groove as the **anterolateral ascending branch**
  - Enters humeral head at junction of greater tuberosity and biceps groove; intraosseous vessel is the **arcuate artery**

3. Posterior humeral circumflex artery
  - Originates from posterior aspect of axillary artery and accompanies axillary nerve inferior to subscapularis muscle to enter quadrilateral space
  - Divides into anterior and posterior branches
  - Anterior branch travels with axillary nerve to supply anterior 2/3 of deltoid and skin overlying mid-deltoid.

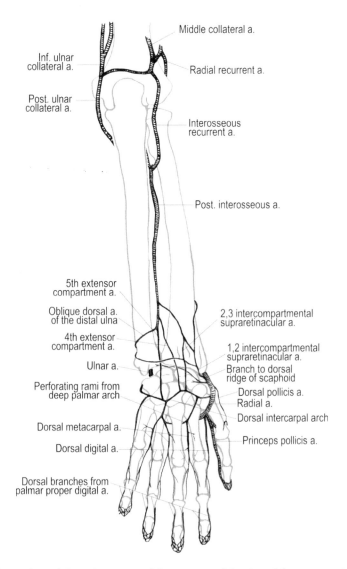

FIGURE 6.2 Illustration of the primary arterial anatomy of the dorsal forearm, wrist, and hand.

BRACHIAL ARTERY

- Continuation of the axillary artery at the inferior border of the teres major muscle
- The **profunda brachii artery** arises posteromedially, just distal to the teres major muscle. The artery courses laterally between the medial and lateral heads of the triceps brachii muscle before piercing the lateral intermuscular septum. It descends between the brachioradialis and brachialis muscles to the region of the lateral epicondyle where it anastomoses with the **radial recurrent artery**.
- The brachial artery is **medial to the median nerve in the upper arm; in the mid-upper arm the relationship changes and the artery courses lateral to the median nerve and medial to the biceps muscle.**
- The brachial artery descends medial to the biceps muscle and is **medial to the biceps tendon** in the antecubital fossa.
- Major branches include:
  - Superior ulnar collateral artery
  - Inferior ulnar collateral artery
  - Radial artery
  - Ulnar artery

VASCULAR SUPPLY OF THE ELBOW

- **Inferior ulnar collateral artery**
  - Branch from brachial artery
  - Penetrates the medial intermuscular septum just proximal to the medial epicondyle to supply the ulnar nerve
  - Anastomosis with anterior ulnar recurrent artery
- **Superior ulnar collateral artery**
  - Branch from brachial artery within the proximal arm
  - Travels distally with the ulnar nerve toward elbow
  - Anastomosis with posterior ulnar recurrent artery
- **Medial collateral artery**
  - Anastomosis with interosseous recurrent artery
- **Radial collateral artery**
  - Anastomosis with radial recurrent artery
  - Penetrates lateral intermuscular septum
- **Radial recurrent artery**
  - Variable origin; may arise from brachial artery or from radial artery

■ *Clinical Correlate:* Anconeus flap—the anconeus muscle is supplied by three arterial pedicles: (i) recurrent posterior interosseous artery; (ii) medial collateral artery; (iii) posterior branch of the radial collateral artery. The first two are present most reliably. Typically, the flap is based on the medial collateral artery.

RADIAL ARTERY (Figs. 6-3 and 6-4)

- Located in the brachioradialis—flexor carpi radialis (FCR) interval in the distal forearm
- Divides into:
  - **Superficial/palmar branch**—courses volar to the FCR tendon and either through or volar to the thenar musculature to contribute to the superficial palmar arch (~36%).
  - **Deep/dorsal branch**
    - Passes deep to the abductor pollicis longus (APL) and extensor pollicis brevis (EPB) tendons at the anatomic snuffbox
    - Overlies the scaphoid-trapezial-trapezoid (STT) joint

- Splits the two heads of the first dorsal interosseous muscle
- Classically terminates through its contribution to the deep palmar arch.

ULNAR ARTERY

- Enters the proximal forearm **deep to the deep head of the pronator teres**
- Remains **radial or lateral to the ulnar nerve** in the forearm and at the distal ulnar tunnel or Guyon's canal.
- Passes **ulnar to the hook of the hamate**
- Terminates as:
  - Volar carpal branch
  - Contribution to superficial palmar arch
  - Contribution to deep palmar arch

MEDIAN ARTERY (ANOMALOUS—PERSISTING)

- Present in approximately 10% to 15%
- Descends with the median nerve through the forearm to the wrist and carpal tunnel; pathology of the persisting median artery may be an etiology of carpal tunnel syndrome

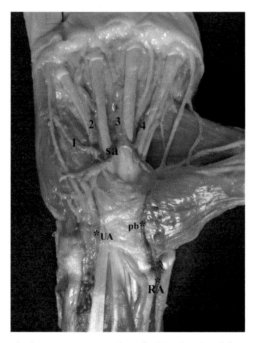

FIGURE 6.3 The radial and ulnar arteries are identified in the distal forearm. The radial artery *(RA)* divides into a deep branch *(>>)* and a palmar branch *(pb)*. The deep branch passes deep to the first dorsal extensor compartment tendons at the anatomic snuffbox, enters the interval between the two heads of the first dorsal interosseous muscle to then divide into the princeps pollicis artery and a branch to the deep palmar arterial arch. The palmar branch courses volar to the FCR tendon (**see Fig. 6-4**) and penetrates the thenar musculature to contribute to the superficial palmar arterial arch *(sa)*. The ulnar artery *(UA)* exits the distal ulnar tunnel and contributes to the superficial palmar arterial arch *(sa)*. The common palmar digital arteries *(1–4)* and the proper ulnar digital artery to the small finger typically originate from the *sa*. In this dissection, the proper ulnar digital artery to the small finger *(1)* arises from the common digital artery to the ring-small interval. Note the location of the *sa* relative to the distal aspect of the transverse carpal ligament and its palmar location relative to the extrinsic digital flexor tendons.

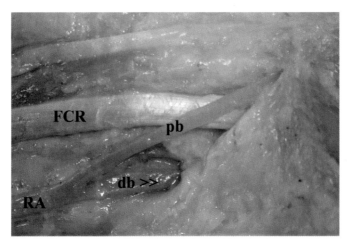

FIGURE 6.4 The intimacy of the palmar branch of the radial artery *(pb)* to the flexor carpi radialis tendon *(FCR)* immediately proximal to the volar wrist crease is relevant to the surgical approach to the volar wrist and distal forearm. The deep branch of the radial artery *(db≫)* is identified as it courses deep to the first dorsal extensor compartment at the radial wrist. Radial artery *(RA)*.

SUPERFICIAL PALMAR ARCH

- **Complete versus incomplete**: a "complete" arch is where an anastomosis is identified between the vessels that constitute the arch.
- **Complete arch (84%)**
  - Type A: 36% (most common); anastomosis between the ulnar artery and palmar branch of the radial artery (branch from radial artery that passes through or superficial to the abductor pollicis brevis [APB] muscle)
  - Type B: (31%) involves ulnar artery only with formation of common digital arteries to the thumb and index web
  - Type C: (13%) anastomosis between persisting median and ulnar arteries
  - Type D: (2%) contributions from persisting median, radial, and ulnar arteries
  - Type E: (2%) branch of the deep arch communicates with ulnar artery–dependent superficial arch
- **Incomplete arch (16%)**
  - Type F: (11%) ulnar artery contributes to entire superficial arch but not to the thumb and index finger
  - Type G: (4%) palmar branch of the radial artery and ulnar artery both contribute to digital perfusion; however, there is no anastomosis between them
- Superficial to the median nerve
- Located approximately 12 mm distal to the carpal tunnel
- Origin of common palmar digital arteries and the proper digital artery to the ulnar side of the small finger
- Common digital arteries then divide into proper digital arteries that continue along the radial or ulnar side of the digit.
- Common digital arteries divide proximal to the division of the common digital nerves.
- *Common digital nerves* are dorsal to the superficial palmar arch and palmar to the flexor tendons in the palm.
- The *proper digital nerves* become palmar to the digital arteries at the level of the metacarpal necks and continue this relationship into the fingers.

DEEP PALMAR ARCH (Figs. 6-5 and 6-6)

- Complete arch with deep or dorsal branch of the radial artery (**distal to its passage through the two heads of the first dorsal interosseous muscle**) and inferior or superior deep branch of ulnar artery. Typically, the radial artery is dominant.
- Proximal to superficial arch
- Typically provides vascular supply to the thumb and to the radial aspect of the index finger via:
  - **Princeps pollicis artery to thumb**
  - **Proper digital artery to radial index finger**
- Palmar metacarpal arteries join the palmar digital arteries at the level of the MCP joints, proximal to the bifurcation of the proper digital arteries.

■ *Clinical Correlate:* A superficial laceration in the palm may transect common palmar digital arteries without compromising the vascularity of the digits due to sufficient vascular supply from the palmar metacarpal arteries.

VASCULAR SUPPLY OF THE CARPUS

- Supplied by branches from the dorsal and palmar carpal arches
  - **Dorsal carpal arches**: radiocarpal, intercarpal, and basal metacarpal transverse arches
  - **Palmar carpal arches**: palmar radiocarpal, intercarpal, and deep palmar arches
- Dorsal arterial network varies; primarily from dorsal carpal branch of the radial artery, arising over the dorsal trapezium

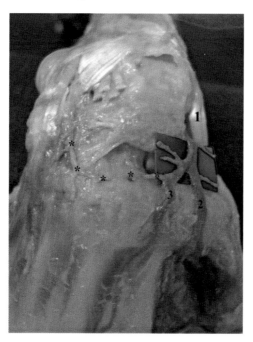

FIGURE 6.5 The emergence of the deep branch of the radial artery at the dorsal wrist from its course deep to the first dorsal extensor tendons *(1)* and its terminal branches. The princeps pollicis artery *(2)* is identified as it descends distally between the two heads of the first dorsal interosseous muscle within the first webspace. The dorsal intermetacarpal artery is seen within the index-long interspace *(3)*. A complete dorsal intercarpal arch is traced *(*****)*. The extensor tendons have been resected at the level of the extensor retinaculum.

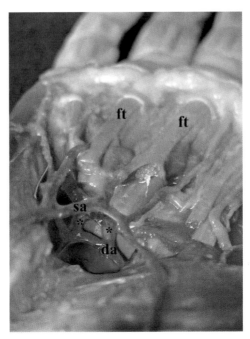

FIGURE 6.6 This oblique view of the wrist highlights the three-dimensional orientation of the superficial palmar arterial arch *(sa)* and the deep palmar arterial arch *(da)*. The median nerve and flexor tendons *(ft)* (cut) have been resected at the wrist in order to illustrate the vascular arches. The deep arch, which is palmar to the carpus, is proximal to the superficial arch that is palmar to the contents of the carpal canal; the two arterial arches are completed by vertically orientated (dorsal-palmar) branches *(^)*.

- **Scaphoid**
  - Primary blood supply (> 70%) is from a branch of the radial artery in the radial snuffbox that supplies the dorsal ridge of the scaphoid.
  - Intraosseous vessels supply the proximal scaphoid pole via retrograde flow.
  - Distal scaphoid pole is supplied by a palmar vascular supply from the radial artery.

■ *Clinical Correlate:* A vascular necrosis of the proximal pole of the scaphoid is due to the interruption of its retrograde intraosseous blood supply.
- **Lunate**
  - Nutrient arteries: 80% from palmar + dorsal vessels; 20% from palmar vessels only.

VASCULAR SUPPLY OF THE DISTAL RADIUS

- Constant vessels include:
  - Radial artery, ulnar artery
  - Anterior interosseous artery (AIA), posterior interosseous artery (PIA)
  - 1,2 intercompartmental supraretinacular artery and 2,3 intercompartmental supraretinacular artery

■ *Clinical Correlate:* The 1,2 intracompartmental supraretinacular artery is used for vascularized bone grafts for the treatment of scaphoid nonunions.
- Fourth and fifth extracompartmental arteries (on extensor surface)

■ *Clinical Correlate:* Vascularized bone grafting to the lunate for treatment of Kienbock disease may utilize the fourth and fifth extensor compartmental artery.

DIGITAL ARTERIAL SUPPLY (Figs. 6-7 to 6-9)

- All five digits receive arterial inflow at the level of the common and/or proper digital artery from **both** the deep and superficial arches in majority of limbs.
- **Three palmar common digital arteries** at the level of the MCP joint have been reported in all studies of arterial variations.
- Proper digital arteries may arise directly from the palmar arches or divide from the common digital arteries to travel along the radial and ulnar aspects of each digit. The arteries are located dorsal and slightly lateral to the digital nerves.
- In general, proper digital arterial dominance has been observed:
  - **Thumb + index (± long):   ulnar > radial**
  - **Ring and small: radial > ulnar**
- Unlike the fingers, the thumb has both an **independent dorsal and palmar arterial supply**, consistently perfused by four vessels: palmar ulnar, palmar radial, dorsal ulnar, and dorsal radial.
- Dorsal thumb perfusion most often arises from the deep branch of the radial artery, prior to its penetration through the muscular bellies of the first dorsal interosseous.
- Palmar perfusion of the thumb classically arises from the **princeps pollicis artery**, the first of four palmar metacarpal arteries, and typically a branch of the deep palmar arch.
- The **radialis indicis artery** (supplies radial aspect of index finger) may originate from the princeps pollicis artery (approximately 50%) or from the deep palmar arch.
- **Vinculum tendinea** are thin, multivessel mesotenon vascular networks that provide a source of tendon nutrition to the dorsal flexor tendons within the digital flexor sheath.
  - **Vinculum longum profundus (VLP)**
  - **Vinculum longum superficialis (VLS)**

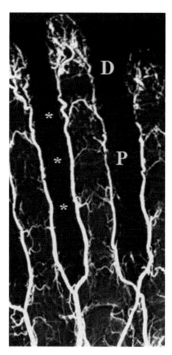

FIGURE 6.7 Arterial perfusion of the long finger demonstrating the transversely oriented "ladder" branches arising from the digital arteries (*). The proximal interphalangeal (P) and distal interphalangeal (D) joints are noted for reference.

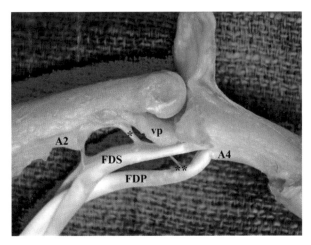

FIGURE 6.8 The vincula tendinum provides a source of nutrition for the digital flexor tendons. The vincula originate from the transverse digital arteries and enter the dorsal surface of the flexor tendons. Here, the flexor digitorum superficialis *(FDS)* and flexor digitorum profundus *(FDP)* tendons have been pulled out from the proximal digital sheath and the *A2* pulley and left within the distal sheath and *A4* pulley to demonstrate the vertically orientated vincular structures. The vinculum brevis superficialis, VBS, *(*)* and the vinculum longus profundus, VLP, *(**)* originate from the proximal transverse digital artery that runs at the level of the A2–A3 interval at the neck of the proximal phalanx. The volar plate of the proximal interphalangeal joint is identified for reference *(vp)*.

- **Vinculum brevis profundus (VBP)**
- **Vinculum brevis superficialis (VBS)**
- **Transverse digital arteries** (digital arterial "ladder branches"):
  - Proximal transverse digital artery is located between A2 and A3 and supplies VBS and VLP.
  - Interphalangeal transverse digital artery is located between A3 and A4 and supplies VBP.
  - Distal transverse digital artery is located between A4 and A5 and supplies VBP.
- The flexor digitorum profundus (FDP) tendon receives blood supply from vessels of intraosseous origin at its insertion at the distal phalanx.

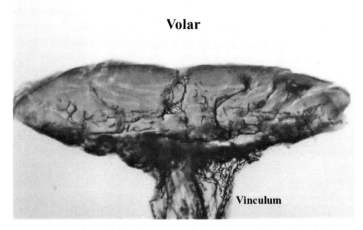

FIGURE 6.9 Transverse section of the intrasynovial portion of the digital flexor tendon (clarified following India ink arterial injection) demonstrating the dorsal vinculum, or mesotenon. The vinculum arises from the digital arterial "ladder" branches and contributes to the nutritional supply of the dorsal flexor tendon.

RECOMMENDED READING

Andary JL, Petersen SA. The vascular anatomy of the glenohumeral capsule and ligaments: an anatomic study. *J Bone Joint Surg.* 2002;84A:2258–2265.

Azar CA, Culver JE, Fleegler EJ. Blood supply of the flexor pollicis longus tendon. *J Hand Surg Am.* 1983;8:471–475.

Coleman SS, Anson BJ. Arterial patterns in the hand based upon a study of 650 specimens. *Surg Gynecol Obstet.* 1961;113:409–424.

Freedman DM, Botte MJ, Gelberman RH. Vascularity of the carpus. *Clin Orthop Relat Res.* 2001;383:47–59.

Gelberman RH, Panagis JS, Taleisnik J, et al. The arterial anatomy of the human carpus, part I: the extraosseous vascularity. *J Hand Surg Am.* 1983;8:367–375.

Gellman H, Botte MJ, Shankwiler J, et al. Arterial patterns of the deep and superficial palmar arches. *Clin Orthop Relat Res.* 2001;383:41–46.

Gerber C, Schneeberger AG, Vinh TS. The arterial vascularization of the humeral head. *J Bone Joint Surg.* 1990;72A:1486–1494.

Hergenroeder PT, Gelberman RH, Akeson WH. The vascularity of the flexor pollicis longus tendon. *Clin Orthop Relat Res.* 1982;162:298–303.

Ikeda A, Ugawa A, Kazihara Y, et al. Arterial patterns in the hand based on a three-dimensional analysis of 220 cadaver hands. *J Hand Surg.* 1988;13A:501–509.

Kleinert JM, Fleming SG, Abel CS, et al. Radial and ulnar artery dominance in normal digits. *J Hand Surg.* 1989;14A:504–508.

Leversedge FJ, Casey PJ, Payne SH, et al. Vascular anatomy of the brachioradialis rotational musculocutaneous flap. *J Hand Surg.* 2001;26A:711–721.

Leversedge FJ, Ditsios K, Goldfarb CA, et al. Vascular anatomy of the human digitorum profundus tendon insertion. *J Hand Surg.* 2002;27A:806–812.

Mestdagh H, Bailleul JP, Chambon JP, et al. The dorsal arterial network of the wrist with reference to the blood supply of the carpal bones. *Acta Morphol Neerl Scand.* 1979;17:73–80.

Moran SL, Cooney WP, Berger RA, et al. The use of the 4 + 5 extensor compartmental vascularized bone graft for the treatment of Kienbock's disease. *J Hand Surg.* 2005;30A:50–58.

Ochiai N, Matsui T, Miyaji N, et al. Vascular anatomy of flexor tendons. I. Vincular system and blood supply of the profundus tendon in the digital sheath. *J Hand Surg Am.* 1979;4:321–330.

Omokowa S, Tanaka Y, Ryu J, et al. Anatomy of the ulnar artery as it relates to the transverse carpal ligament. *J Hand Surg.* 2002;27A:101–104.

Panagis JS, Gelberman RH, Taleisnik J, et al. The arterial anatomy of the human carpus, part II: the intraosseous vascularity. *J Hand Surg Am.* 1983;8:375–382.

Parks BJ, Arbelaez J, Horner RL. Medical and surgical importance of the arterial blood supply of the thumb. *J Hand Surg.* 1978;3A:383–385.

Parry SW, Ward JW, Mathes SJ. Vascular anatomy of the upper extremity muscles. *Plast Reconstr Surg.* 1988;81:358–365.

Schmidt CC, Kohut GN, Greenberg JA, et al. The anconeus muscle flap: its anatomy and clinical application. *J Hand Surg.* 1999;24A:359–369.

Trager S, Pignataro M, Anderson J, et al. Color flow Doppler: imaging the upper extremity. *J Hand Surg.* 1993;18A:621–625.

Yamaguchi K, Sweet FA, Bindra R, et al. The extraosseous and intraosseous arterial anatomy of the adult elbow. *J Bone Joint Surg.* 1997;79A:1653–1662.

Zaidemberg C, Siebert JW, Angrigiani C. A new vascularized bone graft for scaphoid non-union. *J Hand Surg.* 1991;16A:474–478.

Appendix I: Muscle Origins and Insertions

MUSCLE	ORIGIN	INSERTION	INNERVATION	
Abductor pollicis longus	Proximal and dorsal radius and ulna + interosseous membrane	Radial base of thumb metacarpal + thenar fascia	Posterior interosseous nerve	C5, 6, 7, 8
Adductor pollicis	Palmar aspect of long finger metacarpal shaft	Ulnar sesamoid + ulnar base of thumb proximal phalanx + adductor aponeurosis	Deep branch ulnar nerve	C8, T1
Anconeus	Posterior aspect, lateral epicondyle of distal humerus	Proximal ulna, posterior to ECU	Radial nerve	C5, 6, 7, 8
Biceps brachii	Long head at supraglenoid tubercle, short head at anterior lateral coracoid process	Radial tuberosity and bicipital aponeurosis	Musculocutaneous nerve	C5, 6, 7
Brachialis	Anterior aspect of distal humerus	Ulnar tuberosity of proximal ulna	Musculocutaneous + radial nerves	C5, 6, 7
Brachioradialis	Lateral supracondylar ridge of distal humerus	Distal radius, at base of first dorsal compartment	Radial nerve	C5, 6, 7, 8
Coracobrachialis	Lateral inferior aspect of coracoid process of scapula	Medial aspect of middle 1/3 humeral shaft	Musculocutaneous nerve	C5, 6, 7
Deltoid	Lateral anterior clavicle, AC joint, acromion and scapular spine	Deltoid tuberosity of lateral humerus	Axillary nerve	C5, 6
Extensor carpi radialis brevis	Lateral epicondyle of distal humerus	Radial and dorsal aspect of long finger metacarpal base	Radial nerve or posterior interosseous nerve	C5, 6, 7, 8
Extensor carpi radialis longus	Lateral supracondylar ridge of distal humerus, inferior to BR origin	Radial and dorsal aspect of index finger metacarpal base	Radial nerve	C5, 6, 7, 8
Extensor carpi ulnaris	Common extensor tendon from posterior lateral distal humerus	Dorsal and ulnar base of small finger metacarpal	Posterior interosseous nerve	C5, 6, 7, 8

MUSCLE	ORIGIN	INSERTION	INNERVATION	
Extensor digiti quinti	Common extensor tendon from posterior lateral distal humerus	(1) Dorsal base of middle phalanx via central slip; (2) dorsal base of distal phalanx via lateral bands	Posterior interosseous nerve	C5, 6, 7, 8
Extensor digitorum communis	Common extensor tendon from posterior lateral distal humerus	(1) Dorsal base of middle phalanx via central slip; (2) dorsal base of distal phalanx via lateral bands	Posterior interosseous nerve	C5, 6, 7, 8
Extensor indicis proprius	Posterior distal ulna and interosseous membrane	(1) Dorsal base of middle phalanx via central slip; (2) dorsal base of distal phalanx via lateral bands	Posterior interosseous nerve	C5, 6, 7, 8
Extensor pollicis brevis	Distal dorsal radius and interosseous membrane	Dorsal base of thumb proximal phalanx	Posterior interosseous nerve	C5, 6, 7, 8
Extensor pollicis longus	Posterior superior ulna and interosseous membrane	Dorsal base of thumb distal phalanx	Posterior interosseous nerve	C5, 6, 7, 8
Flexor carpi radialis	Anterior medial aspect of medial epicondyle	Radial and palmar base of index finger metacarpal + palmar base of long finger metacarpal	Median nerve	C6, 7, 8, T1
Flexor carpi ulnaris	Anterior medial aspect of medial epicondyle	Pisiform + piso-hamate ligament + pisometacarpal ligament	Ulnar nerve	C8, T1
Flexor digitorum profundus	Anterior interosseous membrane and anterior ulna	Palmar base of distal phalages of index, long, ring, and small fingers	Anterior interosseous nerve (radial half) and ulnar nerve (ulnar half)	C6, 7, 8, T1
Flexor digitorum superficialis	Anterior proximal ulna + interosseous membrane + anterior proximal radius + medial epicondyle	Middle 3/5 of middle phalanges index, middle, ring, and small fingers	Median nerve	C6, 7, 8, T1
Flexor pollicis longus	Anterior interosseous membrane + anterior radius	Palmar base of thumb distal phalanx	Anterior interosseous nerve	C6, 7, 8, T1

MUSCLE	ORIGIN	INSERTION	INNERVATION	
Hypothenar: Abductor digiti quinti	Palmar pisiform + pisohamate ligament	Ulnar base of small finger proximal phalanx + small finger ulnar lateral band	Ulnar nerve	C8, T1
Hypothenar: Flexor digiti quinti	Hook of hamate + TCL	Ulnar base of small finger proximal phalanx	Ulnar nerve	C8, T1
Hypothenar: Opponens digiti quinti	Hook of hamate	Ulnar shaft small metacarpal	Ulnar nerve	C8, T1
Infraspinatus	Infraspinous fossa of posterior scapula	Rotator cuff, middle greater tuberosity of proximal humerus	Suprascapular nerve	C5, 6
Interosseous, dorsal—first	Ulnar and dorsal aspect of thumb metacarpal + radial and dorsal aspect of index finger metacarpal	Radial base of index finger proximal phalanx	Deep branch ulnar nerve	C8, T1
Interosseous, dorsal—second	Ulnar and dorsal aspect of index finger metacarpal + radial and dorsal aspect of long finger metacarpal	Deep head: radial base of long finger proximal phalanx; Superficial head: radial lateral band	Deep branch ulnar nerve	C8, T1
Interosseous, dorsal—third	Ulnar and dorsal aspect of long finger metacarpal + radial and dorsal aspect of ring finger metacarpal	Deep head: ulnar base of long finger proximal phalanx; Superficial head: ulnar lateral band	Deep branch ulnar nerve	C8, T1
Interosseous, dorsal—fourth	Ulnar and dorsal aspect of ring finger metacarpal + radial and dorsal aspect of small finger metacarpal	Deep head: ulnar base of ring finger proximal phalanx; Superficial head: ulnar lateral band	Deep branch ulnar nerve	C8, T1
Interosseous, palmar—first	Ulnar and volar shaft of index finger metacarpal	Ulnar base of index finger proximal phalanx + ulnar lateral band	Deep branch ulnar nerve	C8, T1
Interosseous, palmar—second	Radial and volar shaft of ring finger metacarpal	Radial base of ring finger proximal phalanx + radial lateral band	Deep branch ulnar nerve	C8, T1
Interosseous, palmar—third	Radial and volar shaft of small finger metacarpal	Radial base of small finger proximal phalanx + radial lateral band	Deep branch ulnar nerve	C8, T1

MUSCLE	ORIGIN	INSERTION	INNERVATION	
Latissimus dorsi	Pelvis, spinous processes T7 to T12, thoracolumbar fascia, inferior angle of scapula and ribs 9 to 12	Posterior and medial aspect of proximal humeral shaft, anterior to Teres Major	Thoracodorsal nerve	C6, 7
Levator scapuli	Transverse processes T1 to T4	Transverse processes C1 to C4	Dorsal scapular nerve	C5
Lumbrical— index finger	Radial aspect index FDP tendon, Zone 3	Radial lateral band index finger	Median nerve (from common digital nerve)	C6, 7, 8, T1
Lumbrical— middle finger	Radial aspect middle FDP tendon, Zone 3	Radial lateral band middle finger	Median nerve (from common digital nerve)	C6, 7, 8, T1
Lumbrical— ring finger	Ulnar aspect middle FDP tendon, Zone 3, and radial aspect ring FDP tendon, Zone 3	Radial lateral band ring finger	Deep branch ulnar nerve	C8, T1
Lumbrical— small finger	Ulnar aspect ring FDP tendon, Zone 3, and radial aspect small FDP tendon, Zone 3	Radial lateral band small finger	Deep branch ulnar nerve	C8, T1
Palmaris longus	Anterior medial aspect of medial epicondyle	Palmar fascia/ aponeurosis	Median nerve	C6, 7, 8, T1
Pectoralis major	Clavicular head: Anterior medial half clavicle; Sternocostal head: Lateral sternum and proximal medial anterior rectus sheath	Medial proximal humeral shaft, anterior to Latissimus Dorsi	Medial and lateral pectoral nerves	C5, 6, 7, 8, T1
Pectoralis minor	Anterior ribs 3 to 5, lateral to costochondral junctions	Inferior coracoid process	Medial pectoral nerve	C5, 6, 7
Pronator quadratus	Anterior and ulnar distal radius	Ulnar and palmar aspect of distal 1/3 ulna	Anterior interosseous nerve	C6, 7, 8, T1
Pronator teres	Humeral head: Anterior medial aspect of medial epicondyle, medial supracondylar ridge; Ulnar head: Medial border of coronoid process	Radial aspect of middle 1/3 radius	Median nerve	C6, 7, 8, T1
Rhomboids	Rh. Major—spinous processes of C6, C7; Rh. Minor—spinous processes T1 to T4	Posterior medial scapula at and below scapular spine	Dorsal scapular nerve	C5

MUSCLE	ORIGIN	INSERTION	INNERVATION	
Serratus anterior	Chest wall ribs 1 to 9, lateral to pectoralis minor insertion	Anterior medial scapula	Long thoracic nerve	C5, 6, 7
Subscapularis	Subscapular fossa of anterior scapula	Lesser tuberosity of proximal humerus	Upper and lower subscapular nerves	C5, 6
Supinator	Radial aspect of olecranon + lateral epicondyle + annular ligament + radiocapitellar ligament	Proximal volar radius between biceps and pronator teres insertions	Radial nerve (or posterior interosseous nerve)	C5, 6, 7, 8
Supraspinatus	Supraspinous fossa of posterior scapula	Rotator cuff, superior greater tuberosity of proximal humerus	Suprascapular nerve	C5, 6
Teres major	Inferior aspect of posterior border of scapula	Posterior medial proximal humeral shaft	Lower subscapular nerve	C5, 6
Teres minor	Posterior lateral middle third border of scapula	Rotator cuff, inferior greater tuberosity of proximal humerus	Axillary nerve	C5, 6
Thenar: Abductor pollicis brevis	Palmar scaphoid + trapezium + TCL	Radial base of thumb proximal phalanx + MCP joint capsule	Recurrent motor branch median nerve	C6, 7, 8, T1
Thenar: Flexor pollicis brevis	Deep head: palmar capitate + trapezium; Superficial head: TCL	Radial base of thumb proximal phalanx + MCP joint capsule + radial sesamoid	Recurrent motor branch median nerve and deep branch ulnar nerve	C6, 7, 8, T1
Thenar: Opponens pollicis	Trapezium + TCL + CMC joint capsule	Radial aspect of thumb metacarpal diaphysis	Recurrent motor branch median nerve	C6, 7, 8, T1
Trapezius	Occiput, spinous processes C1 to T12	Lateral clavicle posterior to deltoid, AC joint, acromion, spine of scapula	Accessory nerve (CN XI)	n/a
Triceps	Lateral Head: proximal, posterior humeral diaphysis; Medial (deep) Head: distal, posterior humeral diaphysis; Long Head: lateral infraglenoid scapula	Olecranon	Radial nerve	C5, 6, 7, 8

ECU, extensor carpi ulnaris; BR, brachioradialis; TCL, transverse carpal ligament; FDP, flexor digitorum profundus; CMC, carpometacarpal; MCP, metacarpophalangeal; CN, Cranial Nerve; n/a, not applicable.

Appendix II: Compartments of the Upper Extremity

ARM

- Deltoid
  - May have multiple subcompartments
- Anterior compartment
- Posterior compartment

FOREARM

- Dorsal forearm
- Volar forearm
- Mobile wad

HAND

- Thenar compartment
  - May have multiple subcompartments
- Adductor pollicis

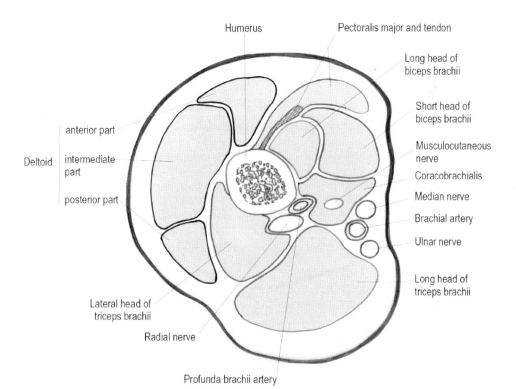

FIGURE AII-1 Transverse section of arm through the upper humeral diaphysis demonstrating the primary osteofascial compartments of the arm.

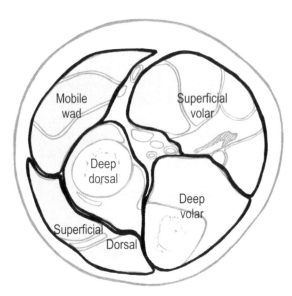

FIGURE AII-2 Cross-section of forearm immediately distal to the biceps tuberosity.

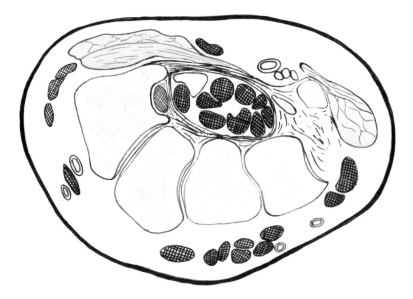

FIGURE AII-3 Cross-section of carpal tunnel at level of distal carpal row.

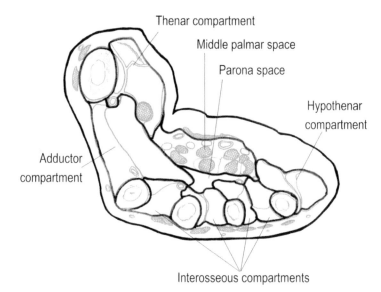

Thenar compartment

Middle palmar space

Parona space

Hypothenar compartment

Adductor compartment

Interosseous compartments

FIGURE AII-4 Cross-section through the base of the hand, distal to the CMC joints, illustrating the multiple osteofascial compartments and palmar spaces.

* Hypothenar compartment
  * May have multiple subcompartments
* Dorsal and volar interosseous muscle compartments
* Carpal tunnel

RECOMMENDED READING

DiFelice A Jr, Seiler JG III, Whitesides TE Jr. The compartments of the hand: an anatomic study. *J Hand Surg.* 1998;23A:682–686.

Gellman H, Buch K. Acute compartment syndrome of the arm. *Hand Clin.* 1998;14:385–389.

Guyton GP, Shearman CM, Saltzman CL. Compartmental divisions of the hand revisited. Rethinking the validity of cadaver infusion experiments. *J Bone Joint Surg.* 2001;83B:241–244.

von Schroeder HP, Botte MJ. Definitions and terminology of compartment syndrome and Volkmann's ischemic contracture of the upper extremity. *Hand Clin.* 1998;14:331–334.

Appendix III: Palmar Spaces of the Hand and Wrist

THENAR SPACE

- Dorsal to the flexor tendons and volar to the interosseous fascia
- **Separated from the midpalmar space by the midpalmar septum**—a fascial septum extending from the palmar fascia to the long finger metacarpal. The thenar space is **radial** to the septum.
- Boundaries—dorsal: adductor pollicis fascia; volar: index flexor sheath + palmar fascia

MIDPALMAR SPACE

- Dorsal to the flexor tendons and volar to the interosseous fascia, separated from the thenar space by the midpalmar septum—a fascial septum extending from the palmar fascia to the long finger metacarpal. The midpalmar space is **ulnar** to the septum.
- Boundaries—dorsal: fascia of second + third volar interosseous; volar: flexor sheaths of long, ring, and small fingers and palmar aponeurosis

HYPOTHENAR SPACE

- Located between the hypothenar septum and hypothenar musculature
- Boundaries—dorsal: periosteum of small metacarpal and deep hypothenar fascia; volar: palmar fascia and fascia of superficial hypothenar muscles

RADIAL BURSA

- Begins at the metacarpophalangeal joint and extends 1 to 2 cm proximal to the transverse carpal ligament
- Typically, the flexor pollicis longus sheath is continuous with the radial bursa

ULNAR BURSA

- Begins at the proximal aspect of the small finger flexor sheath and extends 1 to 2 cm proximal to the transverse carpal ligament
- Small finger synovial sheath may connect with ulnar bursa

PARONA'S SPACE

- Potential space between the flexor digitorum profundus and the pronator quadratus fascia
- Facilitates potential communication between radial + ulnar bursas

■ *Clinical Correlate:* Flexor tendon sheath infection of the thumb or small finger may spread to Parona's space (deep to flexor tendons overlying proximal wrist and pronator quadratus) and continue as horseshoe abscess.

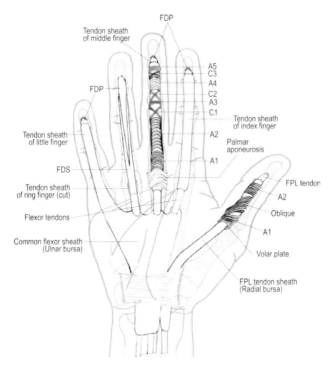

FIGURE AIII-1 Illustration of the palmar spaces of the hand and wrist as well as the digital flexor pulleys.

RECOMMENDED READING

Bojsen-Moller F, Schmidt L. The palmar aponeurosis and the central spaces of the hand. *J Anat*. 1974;117:55–68.

Jebson PJ. Deep subfascial space infections. *Hand Clin*. 1998;14:557–566.

Index

Page numbers followed by the letter *f* refer to figures and letter *t* refer to tables.